Caregiving Tips for Everyone

M. G. Walker

Inspiring Voices®
A Service of **Guideposts**

Inspiring Voices books may be ordered through booksellers or by contacting:

Inspiring Voices
1663 Liberty Drive
Bloomington, IN 47403
www.inspiringvoices.com
1-(866) 697-5313

ISBN: 978-1-4624-0343-1 (sc)
ISBN: 978-1-4624-0342-4 (e)

Library of Congress Control Number: 2012917504

Printed in the United States of America

Inspiring Voices rev. date: 11/2/2012

Contents

Acknowledgements

I would like to thank Jeannie and Tom for their continued support and encouragement during the process of writing this book. My daughter Holly who put up with all the time I spent writing while she helped with the reworking. For Michael who encouraged me to write this book for him and the Doctors, Nurses and Aids both at the Oncology Ward and Clinic, for teaching us so much. And of course to my constant companion Sasha, remaining at the side of those in need until time of us to go.

Preface

This book is set up to help you answer your questions as quickly as possible while you still provide care and take care of yourself during this most important time of your life. The reason for beginning with dementia is that so many illnesses and conditions that affect the elderly or become part of an adult condition have dementia as a component. Dementia can be a very small issue for us on a daily basis; however, when it does rise to the surface, there are ways to accomplish the kind of care that will allow us to get through it easier.

Dementia can be an illness unto itself or it can be a symptom of a condition that has become a predominant part of our lives. Some dementia is easily handled, such as dementia that accompanies dehydration or a medication interaction. These can be taken care of easily and usually very quickly, such as increasing the amount of water a person is drinking. A medication adjustment will require physician involvement, but it will correct itself rather quickly following that adjustment.

Dementia as an illness is an entirely different story and can become overwhelming to deal with. This dementia is with us 24/7 and will impact every aspect of our lives. Most dementias are progressive and will refine your skill in adapting quickly and not missing a beat. This kind of dementia is born from many different illnesses, including Alzheimer's, Parkinson's, mini-strokes, and Huntington's.

Whatever the cause, this book will provide answers to many of your questions and will help you through your day. If you are caregiving to an amputee and cannot imagine how this will help you, check out the chapters on bathing and dressing, loss, or hydration. All of these contain techniques that will help you in your daily routine.

The last dementia is one that arrives and retains the same degree of significance throughout the friend's life. The primary cause of this dementia is brain injury—whether from accident or illness—that injures the brain but leaves no other lasting effects.

This one word can strike fear in the lives of most modern families, but you can meet dementia on its own ground and survive. There are many ways to cope, work, or survive a loved one's diagnosis. Many Americans struggle to cope with caregiving after this diagnosis. Building a new set of coping skills for this intrusion in their lives appears insurmountable. A few short years ago, the answer was professional help in the form of skilled nursing facilities or live-in help. Today's economic setting makes this an issue that needs to be tackled within the family setting.

The solution is here and can be obtained very

quickly with little to no financial burden. You can learn how to cope and live far less stressfully after hearing this diagnosis for a family member. The truth about dementia is in the diagnosis, which can cause dementia. That's right—dementia is stressful for patients and caregivers; as such, it is one of the causations of dementia.

Stress is a cause of dementia. It can be overwhelming. Dementia can be daunting and destructive. Medication, if not managed correctly, can cause dementia. Hydration, if not properly achieved during extreme temperature changes, can cause dementia.

I will show you how to begin your life living with a loved one having dementia. Your survival and possible growth for a stress-less, purposeful life will begin without any new economic expenditure.

You do not need any special tools or degrees. You have all the tools and information you need to work with someone who has dementia. The first—and most important—thing to do is set up a one-hour break for yourself each day during the first month of caring for a person with dementia. This break is *your* time. Do not bring any thoughts of your life maintenance (paying bills, calling back business associates, calling family, cleaning, scheduling auto maintenance, and so forth) into *your* time. Use *your* time for you. Give yourself a break, go for a walk, take a forty-five-minute nap, have a cup tea, coffee, or other nonalcoholic beverage, spend time with a pet, garden, look at a sunset with a clear mind. There are so many more ways to spend *your* time—just sit back and have a focal point of a beautiful picture.

Keep a journal of the highs and lows associated with your loved ones moods and achievements. Watch with interest how your person's daily routine is set up—not by you but by the person you are caring for. When do they get up (on their own without intrusion)? When do they go to bed (again without intrusion)? How have they set up their personal hygiene rituals? What are their personal eating rituals? How do they spend their quality time? What other activities make up each day of their life?

Caring for a person with dementia is very different from any other caregiving. Dementia does not have bandages, ointments, or (in many cases) visible wounds. The number one thing you must remember for having a successful role in this person's life is you are there by their invitation—and they must always be treated this way. Every day is a new adventure in caregiving.

This book is set up to give you an opportunity to read as much or as little you want to at any specific time. It is set up to give you the opportunity to gather your thoughts and help in a specific area of caregiving. If you are in a hurry or need a quick reference, it will be easily found.

I hope you will get some help and know that the road you have chosen is forged ahead of you, and you will be able to shed light for those coming up behind you.

Chapter 1:

What Is a Caregiver?

You must know that *you* are the greatest resource your friend has. Let's be clear; when I say "friend," this references your family member, your friend, your client, your patient, or whatever name you wish to use for the fortunate person you care for. The person you care for is a friend on one level or another. You must keep this in mind as you go through the daily task of walking beside him or her. This is another point I want you to know: we walk *beside* this person—never in front or behind. The journey is theirs; we only provide the help along the way.

One of the keys to being a good caregiver is taking care of yourself. As we provide for our friend, we tend to forget about our own needs. If we take care of ourselves, we will be there for our friend all along this journey we have embarked upon. It is so easy to lose sight of our own lives and needs while providing for a friend who cannot at this minute take care for himself or herself.

You will need to help others give you a break. Asking someone to help is a good beginning, but you might want to provide an experience for your friend as well. Many assisted-living and skilled-nursing facilities (SNF) offer respite care. Not all of us can afford this despite the very reasonable prices.

When someone asks, "What should I get you or your friend for Christmas?" you can respond with the name of an environment or a setting you have found that meets your friend's needs. The respite can be for a few hours or an overnight visit. This will give both of you a much-deserved break.

Please take a few moments and plan ahead for a break. Using a canvas grocery bag or similar item, place things you would take if someone walked through the door and said, "You have four hours. Go be free." You can take a book, a coupon for a movie theater, a warm wrap, a bottle of water, maybe some lotions and polish to give yourself a manicure, and a few pieces of chocolate. It is important to pack now because, if you get the opportunity, you do not want to think about what you will take.

If the bag is in your car, you might take it out and use it for another reason. That's fine, but you need to replace the items as soon as possible. Maybe you will find something else you want to put in the bag. Try to remember that it cannot be emphasized enough how important it is to take good care of yourself.

Every Day Is a New Adventure

Caregivers everywhere know that each day offers a new picture of the friend they care for. This picture can—and does—run an expressway of highs and lows. The highs can make them laugh, cry, and be the happiest people in the world. The lows can knock them down to the lowest point they have ever been.

Here is the good news. The important lifeline for many caregivers is they can control the ups and downs of caregiving to a great degree. All the emotions of our friend can be mirrors of us. If we, as caregivers, are having a bad day or something has upset us, we must leave this outside the door of our friend's house. When we go to any job in a bad mood, most people around us can tell. When everyone is well in the circle we have entered, people leave us to sort out our own stuff. However, our friend needing care cannot do this. Many times, he or she simply mirrors our frustration.

Activities of Daily Living (ADLs) are everything we do to take care of ourselves each day—from the most private and basic to the most difficult and pub-lic. Because ADLs are so basic, we must attend to them no matter what else is happening. They include brushing our teeth, using the restroom, combing our hair, taking medicine, bathing, and getting dressed.

What can we do when this train is off the track? The most important word in our vocabulary will become *simplify*. We all know that we cannot argue with our friend and win. So we can simplify. "Don't want to take the medicines? Okay." Try leaving that for a little while—say, five minutes—and then give only half of the seven or eight pills this person has to take. Go back a little later—say, another five minutes—and give the rest of the pills. Our friend may say, "These are not all my pills." Agree. Say, "We must have forgotten," and give the friend all of the pills. Let's say our friend does not want to use the restroom. Let go of that thought for a few minutes and then go back as though the first exchange did not happen.

If we must let some ADLs go, how about the ones that are not life sustaining? Trade off medicines for getting dressed. Would it really be so awful if our friend stayed in a robe all day or until noon? Trade off washing hair today for using the restroom. (Each time you come back to the chore, it will be new for our friend. Or at least our friend might not be so frustrated by it.)

At this point, we notice that we are giving some control back to our friend who is losing all control. This is especially important in a skilled-care setting because we have taken even the most private decisions away from our friend. And yes, even with the illness or accident, our friend is still in that same body he or she has always been in. He or she may not be able to express his or her wishes, but we can help. Caregivers carry not only the physical weight of this role, but, almost more importantly, we carry the human role of our friend. We should always remember that and keep this thought front and center in each thing we say and do for our friend.

We should always ask permission to accomplish a task for our friend. As professional caregivers working in a professional setting—nursing home, assisted-living facility, adult family home, or at home—our friend should not be addressed in a familiar term of endearment. These words, although spoken with true caring, can create problems far beyond our mind at the time (honey, dearie, love, Mom, Grandma, and sweetheart). But if our friend really is our mother, grandmother, grandfather, and so forth, then the terms are acceptable.

Have you ever noticed while visiting with your friend that an answer to a question or a question you ask seems out of context or off subject? We all do this from time to time. With all the noise going on around us, our minds wander to what to cook for dinner, whom we need or forgot to call, or how to approach a difficult subject with our friend.

The answer to this can be as simple as being over-stressed by our busy lifestyles (and adding an illness to the daily regimen or caregiving to an already hectic day). It can be difficult if our friend cannot seem to think and put sentences together any longer due to the illness. If this is new or has gotten more pronounced, a medical appointment is in order. However, if it is the natural progression of the illness, this can be one of the most difficult areas of caregiving.

If this is a natural progression, your friend may not understand the situation. If your friend knows the situation, this can—and often does—become the catalyst for many difficult and frustrating times. This frustration may be expressed as anger, weeping, or withdrawal.

We can discuss some tools to help keep things less frustrating and running more smoothly. At this point, it is very important that you get at least one hour of stress relief each day. You can be the most helpful and caring person to your friend by having the ability to look at each situation with fresh eyes.

One tool for conversation is to place the burden of conversation on our friend and ask only short answer questions. "Do you want fish for dinner?" This makes the answer a short yes or no. After the answer, you feel confident you have correctly understood the wishes of your friend. Then you carry on the conversation regarding a fishing trip that you remember or a story your friend likes to hear about fishing.

One process we can use to help move through each day is to look at caregiving as a prosthetic or physical-therapy model (giving support to the worrisome action we want to elicit) and not the medical model that a shot or pill will fix. Using tools to help your friend get through each day with the least amount of frustration will make life far more pleasant for you and your friend.

An excellent tool to help pass time in a constructive way is to look at pictures of trips or parties and reminisce with your friend. Remember to keep answers short and easy when caregiving time seems to be at a premium, especially if the caregiver is a family member. It might seem like a waste of time when your whole day is set on a timeline. However, a few monuments of quality time—even fifteen minutes—can set in motion a far better day for all of us. Try to build in little breaks for yourself so that when you are ready to complete a task and your friend is not, you will be able to take a breath and relax to meet your friend on their ground.

If we can learn to look at a situation and think of the best way our friend would want to get through the situation, our days will be far more pleasant. Communication can be achieved in many ways. When answering verbally is not possible, try watching facial expressions or body language for you cues. Family caregivers are also a blessing. Family usually has some insights that are the greatest tools of all.

Unraveling the Puzzle

If we are new on the scene or not familiar with the early life of our friend, there are many aspects of this life that will be invaluable as we walk beside our friend during their illness. And even in the later stages of a life-threatening illness, we can learn and utilize information about these aspects to help our friend to be more comfortable. Having knowledge of our friend's life—beginning with information—provides us with a blueprint of important passages of time and a patchwork of values.

There are many places to begin the research. First, we can ask family (don't rely solely on any part of the information-gathering process). Family usually has some past knowledge that we can include in our history of our friend. However, do not assume you can get all the answers from family in this age of second, third, or more marriages. Also, this is not a license to pry into our friend's life.

Especially true is the information in multiple marriages when our friend is suffering from Alzheimer's disease. Another facilitator of copious amounts of information is picture albums (many times we find that the first or second spouse has given these to the children of that marriage). The information gained from picture albums is primary to provide employment, social, and emotional history. This may also provide some health history, but it will not be so important in that arena.

Look closely at the pictures—and past the event where they were taken. Is our friend having a good time? Are they happy? Are they taking part in a team game event, social party, or dance? Do you recognize their children in the younger face of our friend or the spouse of our friend? (This is especially important if our friend has a dementia, which robs them of today, and the adult children look like the spouse). This is when we can run into the daughter being mistaken for her mother and our friend's wife or the son being mistaken for the male counterparts.)

Another resource for information regarding our friend is to go to the home where our friend has been living and use a new set of eyes. Are there notes to remind our friend of meetings or appointments? Do we see evidence of a hobby that our friend took special pride in? Can our friend continue this hobby in the current living situation? As you look at this hobby, try to think out of the box regarding how our friend can still enjoy this. (A fisherman may enjoy working on his fishing boat, which is no longer possible, but you might take an eight-foot-by-eight-foot section of fishing net, a small amount of patching products, and some tools so our friend can help repair the netting for his fishing business.)

Another good possibility is talking with old friends. I encourage you to do so and find out all you can. This information will be comforting and will help relax our friend when and if we need to help with emotional issues. It is important to know about traumas and catastrophic events in our friend's life. We certainly do not want to be the catalyst for reliving them, but should the memory came back, there will possibly be a way we can help guide our friend to calmer emotions.

One last thing we will want to have is a clear understanding if our friend says he or she want to go home. Do not assume we know the destination of home. Try to ferret out the home we are talking about. You may be surprised by what our friend means.

Caregiving—Not Controlling

I have seen and heard of times when a caregiver becomes so embroiled in providing care for a person that the caregiver cannot—or does not—have a life outside of this role. This is in many cases when the caregiver takes ownership of all that is said and done for the friend. This is not something that the caregiver sets out to do. In fact, it is the furthest thought from their mind. In truth it is a slow evolution of all parts of the caregiving situation.

In today's economic state, it is very difficult to not get caught up in the economics as well as the mechanics of caregiving. This is especially true for family caregivers—but not for the reasons you may think. This is not a case of being concerned about one's own wellbeing; rather, it is a case of trying to do too much. And all this is packaged with a beautiful bow of love.

It is especially difficult for a husband or wife to live with—and care for—a spouse with a debilitating disease. Although the husband or wife very well may know exactly what their friend would want right down to what time to turn on the TV or start the bath or if the coffee is just right, how can they maintain a relationship that allows for self-care? Frequently, they can't. After all, they have been married for more than forty or fifty years, and the bonds are stronger than life in some cases.

Caregivers don't just wake up one day and decide

they have given all their life to our friend and decides that now it is time to take over. In reality, the slow progression of a disease feeds more and more reliance on the caregiver who is becoming exhausted at the same time. Slowly, the caregiver begins to make decisions because they have been getting the same answer for several months. Why not? Soon that grows to fewer opportunities for our friend to express autonomy and puts more reliance on the caregiver. These changes are subtle and increase over time. They can be unobserved by medical professionals, friends, family, clergy, and paid caregivers.

Then something will happen—usually a crisis—and the house of cards will fall. We would hope the person who sees the problem and comes to the caregiver's aid would be a family member or trusted friend. However, in many cases, the person seeing the problem is in the emergency medical field, and the caregiver sees their attempts at help as interfering in the job most cherished by the caregiver. This usually brings in the members of Adult Protective Services; their presence can be frightening for the caregiver.

It is so important for caregivers to take breaks. Take these half-day or all-day breaks and leave the home to go do something for yourself. Your household chores will get done, and those bills will get paid. You need time to catch your breath. Taking care of yourself is something you have to do for yourself. It allows you to provide the caregiving you want and need to do.

Simplify

Being with our friend and simplifying may seem to be opposites. We can become so overwhelmed with day-to-day living and getting through that simply adjusting to a new aspect is a hurdle to get over.

Simplifying when looking at the ADLs may look hard, but it couldn't be easier. We will accomplish the same result with less work. Let's look at the dressing ordeal. It is hard for our friend who has dressed themselves for the last fifty or so years to have someone else helping them with this task.

The first part is for us to determine what the appropriate dress is for the day. It is very possible we know of an appointment or a visitor that our friend has forgotten. Once we know what the appropriate clothing is, we must determine where our friend is in the process. If there is still some cognitive ability to select the clothing, we will want to honor our friend's decision.

You should place the clothing in front of the closet door. This will be the first item seen by our friend, and it will be more easily accepted. If our friend is past this point, place the clothing on the bed or in a chair for them to select. Remember to make the selections without our friend present. This will help maintain our friend's autonomy and make it easier for both of us.

At some point, our friend will become weaker and need assistance in putting on the clothes. This is difficult because our friend is embarrassed—and we are tired. This is a good time to begin simplifying clothing. Over a period of days or weeks, slowly change out clothing that goes over the head (this can be a challenge for many healthy people). When replacing clothing, select clothing with zippers or Velcro closures.

As our friend needs more and more assistance, gradually substitute looser fitting clothing for more restrictive clothing. An example would be to change out the jeans and khakis for athletic wear. Warm-up suits are great for our friends on two levels: (1) they are easier to put on and (2) they will keep our friend warmer. Now about the shoes—this is an item of safety. We do not want our friend tripping over shoestrings. We can go to Velcro closures on shoes or we can go to a heavy slipper. Whichever is decided upon, we need to be sure of the fit. Walking out of a shoe is just as dangerous as tripping on shoestrings.

At some point, we must get to the topic of underwear. This is another difficult decision that may be upsetting to our friend. We should try to balance a big plate as we make this decision. We do not want to embarrass our friend with an accident in public, but we do not want to cross the bridge to Depends, Assurance, or any of the others before it is necessary. The item should be designed by the manufacturer specifically for the male or female friend we are serving.

We need to decide if it is more appropriate to have

ones that will lay flat and have closures on the sides or ones that pull up. The timing of this decision and style of the garment should be made by you before the article is provided to our friend. I have always found it easier to simply undo the side closure, discard the used garment, and provide the next garment in a standing position in public restrooms than to try to balance my friend and pull up the undergarment.

The most important decision we make is to continue to provide the dignity and respect necessary for our friend to maintain their self-respect. We must respect our friend enough to give them the help they require to maintain their dignity.

Take Time to Breathe

Self-care for caregivers seems contradictory. As a caregiver, one is so busy doing exactly what the work suggests. The work of caregiving goes on for twenty-four hours a day and has been referred to as the thirty-six-hour day (there is also a book with the same title). Who could ever argue with the amount of tasks, lack of time, and more tasks coming up each minute?

No one can argue with this time involvement or inability to take a break. However, you must take breaks and schedule relaxation times to recharge your own batteries. This is vital to your life. Many studies and papers have addressed long-term caregiving's negative effect on human life. One study claims an astounding 25–30 percent of caregivers pass away before the friend they are caring for.

Taking studies, papers, professors, and researchers out of the equation, let's look at the day-to-day operation. As the caregiver, if we become ill with the flu, we won't want to pass it on to our friend. What will happen to our friend? The death rate among caregivers with other health restrictions is markedly higher than those without health restrictions. If our system is rundown, it not only becomes open to opportunistic illness, it also takes much longer to get back up to speed.

If the flu turns to pneumonia, not only are we talking weeks of recovery, but possible hospitalization. Now we really have a problem. Who has been trained to take care of our friend? Where is the safety net? Is it a child that lives out of state or has a job they must make arrangements to take time off from.

All these realistic situations can—and do—come into play when a caregiver becomes ill. The best care you can give during your illness is to take care of yourself. Get the recommended rest and come back to the art of caregiving rested and ready for the next step. There are safety nets in most communities. It is called respite care. Check them out and know how to access them if and when you need them. You will be happy you did.

This is not included to scare you. This is a very real part of our lives. If you are a paid caregiver, where is your backup plan? We know you document information all day and keep track of changes in case of emergencies. We want to identify the nuts and bolts of medications, dosages, times, and pharmacies, doctors, contact information, and schedules. Which foods are especially well liked? Is there a special diet or texture? As a paid caregiver, your first allegiance is to your patient.

Notes

Chapter 2:

Activities of Daily Living

Activities of Daily Living (ADLs) are basically a system to provide information about where and how our friend needs help to exist without another person doing for them. The first and arguably most important one is whether our friend can distinguish between a life-threatening emergency and a nonemergency. Once this is determined, can our friend access help without prompting? In order for a person to accomplish this task adequately, they must know what an emergency is, how to access the necessary help, and be capable of repeating the necessary information to obtain the help (type of emergency, address and phone number, and who is in the home) and follow the basic directions given by the other person on the phone. The last may be the most difficult because there is the need to follow directions from an inanimate object (not a person standing in front of them).

Typically, these activities are not activities as in playing a game or watching TV; these activities facilitate our normal daily routines, such as eating, bathing, and showering. Our friend would accomplish these activities on their own if possible. It is extremely important for the caregiver to remember that the accomplishment of these activities are our friend's accomplishment to their liking and possibly will not match ours. If our friend does not want to eat three basic meals a day, but would prefer to graze throughout the afternoon—and a nutritionist has found no harm will be done by eating in this manner—let our friend meet their nutritional needs in this manner. With that said, all of these activities must be accomplished for our friend to have a safe and whole life.

It is especially important to keep in mind we are the facilitator of the ADL and not the provider. Let our friend do as much as possible for themselves. This is so important to provide for their autonomy. When looking at the pattern of ADLs, it is very important that we stick to the timeline that has been our friend's lifetime ritual as much as possible. For example, our friend has showered in the morning four days a week for all of their adult life. We should not now attempt to make a routine of bathing in the evening. If our friend has stayed up late much of their adult life and slept in until 9:00 or 10:00, now is not the time to begin trying to get them up at 6:00 or 7:00 just because that will meet our daily cleaning routine.

We are here to support our friend—not to mother them or medically treat them. Begin by learning the schedule. By following it as closely as possible, we will have far less backlash when trying to accomplish the task at hand. Many establishments have an activity or ADL calendar. Set up a working calendar—with a list of personal needs listed by time and day—and be sure to place it in a convenient area.

- 8:00   Get out of bed, go to the toilet, wash hands
- 9:00   Eat breakfast
- 10:00   Brush teeth, comb hair, put on clothes
- 11:00   Go to the toilet
- Noon   Eat lunch
- 1:00   Go for a walk (even if only in the house), get exercise
- 2:00   Activity of choice (Read, TV, listen to music, and so on)
- 3:30   Take a short rest
- 5:00   Get ready for dinner (go to toilet, wash hands, comb hair, go sit at table)
- 6:00   Eat dinner
- 7:00   Help with dinner clean up, sit and have brief conversation with us
- 8:00   Get ready for bed (brush teeth, change clothes, put away anything left out from afternoon activity)
- 9:00   Get in bed

Of course, this is only an example. Medications will need to be given and accounted for with this plan, as well as any trips out of the house.

Typically, days go smoother when a regimen is followed. However, as a cautionary tale, be sure to leave time for changes. There is nothing like throwing someone's day completely off because they didn't get extra rest or help with a chore. Conversely, we can't keep the house in reasonable order if our friend is having a bad day and is refusing medication.

Mapping will help us with many of the day-to-day challenges we come across. Mapping is easy and will become a tool you, once learned, use frequently. This tool is used to help predict behavior, improve daily routines, and complete some daily tasks.

Mapping is done with a paper and pencil; the only requirement is being able to read and write (no specialized training or degree). Tack up a piece of paper in the kitchen, bathroom, and bedroom. The paper should have date and day of week, morning, noon and night, for column headings, along with one for "concern." Draw lines for the seven days in rows across the paper. Once you have a grid to map out behaviors and concerns, tie the pencil on a string to keep it with the paper. That way, at a moment's notice, you can jot down a quick reference.

Use the map for a month and look at the likes and differences that have occurred which you can control. Maybe our friend's afternoon nap was disrupted by clothes dryer, and they became easily frustrated in the afternoon. As you go through the month, you notice that every time the clothes dryer is used, our friend becomes frustrated in the routine after. This will give us the opportunity to look at the possibility of change, which will make life a bit easier for both of us.

Change is not easy for our friend and probably not for us either. However, if we can have a more peaceful day and week, isn't it worth it? Make small changes at first and wait for the desired result. Continue mapping to have feedback for our benefit. Do not try to change more than one behavior at a time—and remember that Rome was not built in a day.

When our friend becomes frustrated and seems to be losing control, help them by calming down the environment. Give our friend a break from the noise of our world. No loud TV, put a sign on the door for no visitors, do not use bread makers, mixers, and so forth in the kitchen. Sometimes it is hard to believe how much noise is going on around us. There is almost continual stimulation from different noises. All of us can use a break once in a while, and everybody reaches a breaking point with noise at different times.

If our friend is open to suggestions—and you want to try this—it will help. Deep breathing exercises are a great way to minimize the frustration and give added oxygen to our body. Sit in a kitchen chair with a straight back (our friend's chair should have arms for ease of getting up) and take deep breaths that lift our shoulders up with each breath in and down with each breath out. This is an excellent exercise for both of us.

Eating

Caregivers know one of the most important activities is eating. Even if nothing else gets accomplished, eating must occur. This is not always an easy one to accomplish. Should there be an issue with eating, solve the puzzle and get the train back on track. It may sound easy, but it can be very difficult. If our friend is capable of telling us what the problem is or can give us a hint, we are ahead of the game. If we need to start from scratch with little or no insight about the problem, we should begin with the mechanics of eating.

Is our friend wearing dentures? Do the dentures fit correctly? Does our friend have a sore throat or is swallowing a problem? This may require a visit to a speech therapist, which will require a consultation with a physician. In the meantime, use nutritional supplements, milkshakes, and so on. The physician or nurse can give you ideas. However, at each meal between now and the appointment, offer food.

As people age, their sense of taste and smell often decrease. If you stimulate the appetite with small morsels of tasty food, you probably will have more luck within thirty minutes. One mistake we all make is to put too much on the plate for our friend. Our friend's body is not using as much food, and they also have trouble with many items on the plate. Simplify the plate by putting two or three items on the plate. If it appears this is too much, cut one out. When one item is finished, give them another small plate of food. Dinnerware and utensils may also need to be simplified down to one piece of silverware. A small plate with a dark circle around the edge helps our friend differentiate between surfaces and foods. Once you master the technique of unraveling the question, you will do fine. Always keep in mind that we are the facilitator, helping our friend with meeting the goals of the day.

Give our friend plenty of time to eat. Do not hover over them or ask if they are done as soon as they put down the fork. It is preferred to not use any words that could indicate they have finished eating. Instead, you can ask, "Would you like some fruit? How would you like some cobbler? Are you ready for your potatoes?" The elderly tend to not eat enough of a balanced diet; this is when you can balance the meal out.

Always try to have a glass of water on the table in front of our friend. We do not drink enough water and, as a consequence, suffer longer fevers, frequent infections, and more hospitalizations due to dehydration. During mild and hot weather, keep plenty of popsicles, watermelon, grapes, lemonade, and other things with high water content. Frozen fruit can be a nutritious snack, meal, or dessert. It will meet three daily needs: servings of fruit, extra healthy calories, and a new texture that may stimulate hunger for a meal.

Bathing

Learning our friend's preferences and needs is an absolute necessity. Can they still wash themselves if all items are set out and within reach? If so, by all means let them. The caregiver should always be within a door away. Should our friend fall or require help, we must be there at a moment's notice, always making sure to ask permission to enter. (The activity of being right outside while our friend accomplishes their own bathing is called "Stand By.")

There is a ritual that seems to work best regardless of what stage of need our friend is in. Leave our friend to finish coffee or watch TV and place clothing in a space easily reached where our friend will be at the time of dressing. Place clothing in the order that it is put on: briefs/panties, undershirt/bra, socks, pants, shirt/blouse, and sweater or light jacket if necessary. Then do the same for toiletries, always following the same order. At this time, place the bath chair in the shower or tub if it is not already inside.

Move to the bathing order: washcloth, soap, shampoo, conditioner, and towel. Once we have learned the order, the routing will be accomplished easily and quickly.

The next part of this topic is important. When our friend can no longer bathe themselves, but can get on the bath chair by themselves, there is a decision to make. A bath aide can be hired or you can do it. Should this be a task you want or have decided to take on, there are some points you might want to consider.

Do not bring our friend into the bathroom until you have prepared the clothing and bathing tools. Make sure that you have the bath chair in place. Make sure the washcloth and towel are readily available, along with soap, shampoo, and conditioner.

If we must do the mechanics of bathing, there is a specific way to do so that will maintain as much dignity and autonomy as possible. Make sure the bath water is warm to the touch. This will relax our friend and limit the anxiety of taking a shower or bath. Next, get the washcloth wet and soapy, put the washcloth in our friend's hand, and guide the hand so that our friend is doing the bathing. If done appropriately, our hand will never touch our friend. Continue to follow this pattern through the entire bathing process.

Limiting our touching of our friend during this time is extremely important. This allows our friend to feel relaxed and not anxious or frightened. Our friend will begin a pleasant day on a positive note or go to bed for the night and get the appropriate rest.

Bathing and toileting are extremely personal tasks that need the approach of absolute professionalism. Allow our friend to accomplish or help all they want. If our friend indicates they do not want to be touched in a particular area, leave that area and come back to it a little later in the bathing or toileting. If they still do not want to be touched during bathing, let this go for a day and see if the behavior reverses itself. If it does not, it is time to be sure our friend does not have something else going on (UTI, yeast infection, hemorrhoids, etc.). If our friend never wants to have you help with the bathing in the most private areas, try some substitutions. Get baby wipes (these are gentle and have no perfume) or a similar item and let them do their own bathing.

Toileting

This can be quite a difficult issue. If we are a family caregiver, it may be a matter of dignity for our friend. There is also the gender issue for some people. This is a time when we will be able to discuss and move forward if we remember to use the tools we have learned about dignity and privacy.

Keeping in mind the dignity of our friend, it is very acceptable to suggest use of the facilities prior to going out—especially if we are aware of a need to be out for a longer period of time. Medical appointments, dental appointments, hair appointments, shopping, and exercise are all appointments that can take some time.

If there is concern about our friend being able to find the appropriate facility (toilet or sink) after relieving themselves, which can be very embarrassing for our friend, there is a suggestion to help out. When we get older, we can have difficulty seeing. Lighting in bathrooms is not always what it could be. In pastel bathrooms, a contrast of a darker color is very helpful. A darker toilet seat or backsplash on the sink will designate the location of the toilet and sink.

If the situation is such that we need to help our friend out in public, there are growing numbers of family restrooms in many public venues. This can be a difficult situation to handle. It is also permissible to go into the gender-specific restroom and ask another to make certain that anyone wanting to enter is aware that we are providing assistance inside.

Dressing

This activity is easier to grasp for some than others; however, if you can always think of dressing from the skin out, you are in a good place. It will help if the clothing is always placed in the same manner. This is of particular importance if our friend is having attention lapses. It will become second nature to stack the clothes with outer clothing (shirt, pants) on the bottom and undergarments on top. Shoes go last.

Clothing should be easy to get on, easy to remove for toileting or medical appointments, and absorb perspiration. This is especially true if our friend is overweight; try to use 100 percent cotton clothing for them. Cotton will absorb a considerable amount of perspiration. If the outer clothing is sticking to our friend while toileting, get them changed so we do not breed bacteria.

An important part of dressing is keeping an

eye on our friend's skin, especially as their ability to communicate is waning. If they are particularly susceptible to skin breakdown, we should watch for clothing that is binding, too loose, or creates a deep fold mark in the skin. We must take immediately action if this is noted. Discolored, red, or moist skin can become ulcers before you know it. This will create infections; if left untreated, it can lead to death.

Skin breakdown is a very large concern among caregivers. It goes by many names—bedsores, pressure sores, or ulcers—and can appear anywhere on the body. This is one of the reasons for helping our friend dress. If our friend is heavyset, check the skin rolls, under the breasts of men and women, buttocks, heels, backs, and shoulders. These areas hold moisture and frequently have all of our friend's weight on them. Anyone can get skin breakdown; the difference is how soon—and to what degree—it is treated.

Our friend should have good shoes, such as tennis shoes, to protect them from falls. The shoes should have Velcro closures rather than shoestrings. Velcro closures will save us from a shoestring-tying situation and stepping out of the shoes.

Keep in mind our friend does not want to impose on us but cannot help it. This is important for caregivers helping men since they want to take care of us. They feel especially devalued when help is necessary to meet the most basic needs.

Always treat them with the most professional

respect and allow them to do what they are able to help themselves.

Sleeping

Our friend should stick to a bedtime schedule as much as possible. Every effort should be made to keep this schedule and any bedtime routines. Scheduling is very important for maintaining health for our friend. Should the routine change or be nonexistent, everything else in our friend's life will suffer.

The first item on the agenda for good sleep and maintaining a routine is toileting just before bed. Be sure the pathway from the bed to the bathroom is clear of hazards; this will become even more necessary as time goes on. If our friend is sleeping in a room with its own bathroom attached, there are two things that you can do to help provide quality sleep patterns.

- Have a nightlight in the bathroom. Be sure that this is a nice soft white or clear bulb that stays on all the time. There will not be concern on our friend's part regarding the light if this is the case.
- Be sure there is no unnecessary furniture or hazards in this bedroom. Our friend will, undoubtedly, awaken to use the restroom and will be in a hurry. Items in the room may become tripping or falling hazards if they are left in our friend's way.

It is best not to shut our friend's door because, as the illness progresses, people sometimes feel a shut door means they must stay in the room no matter what. Although a chair may seem nice to have in the room, should our friend fall over it or onto it, they could be severely hurt. If our friend cannot find the toilet, they will use other places to meet the need. If, as our friend is working through the disease process, they need grab-bars to get off the toilet and one side of the toilet does not have a place for this rail, take a walker (just the plain aluminum without wheels) and turn it backward, setting it over the toilet. This works well and avoids a home renovation.

Most, if not all, wandering at night can be attributed to looking for the bathroom or being hungry. Both of these triggers can be easily handled with a little forethought. Do not leave food or drink in the bedroom; they can be choking hazards. Instead, leave these items on top of a dresser or just outside the door. Be aware that food and drink in the bedroom will get spilled from time to time. Look at our friend realistically in terms of wandering. If our friend is prone to wandering, let's not encourage this trait.

Remember to wake our friend gently and do not stand over them. This may sound like it can't be done; however, if we don't follow some very careful guidelines, this can be disastrous. When a person first awakens, they may be unaware of who we are or where they are (this is especially true for our friends taking multiple prescriptions as frequently they sleep very soundly). It is best to stand in the doorway and call out to them. This may seem over the top, but for a person whose thoughts are not clear, a person standing over them or touching them is a threat.

Although this threat is a perceived one, it is just as frightening and can have significant results. Try allowing them to wake on their own—this really is best. However, it is frequently not possible. I have found a radio set to a classical music station or a CD with nature sounds is another way to gently wake someone.

Surviving the Seasons

Each season brings a new set of rewards and challenges. We can use this to help break up the activity and daily routine. Change is difficult for some, and this is a way of keeping some change without overwhelming our friend. Change is good because it forces us to use another part of our brain to work out the living situation. Embrace change and keep in mind that a little goes a long way.

Winter

Winter a time to reminisce and renew. Just as seasons carry us through the year, so do these times in our lives. Winter is a time for looking back at the fall or summer and looking forward to what will be. It is easy to become a couch potato in the winter. This is not good for anyone, but especially for us as we age. Our metabolic rate (how we use our food) slows down naturally—and then we add inactivity.

There are activities we can do without leaving the house if the weather is not permitting. However, if we can get out, that is what we should do. Going to a mall or indoor track to walk is a great way to stimulate our muscles and our intellect. Frequently, we will see people we know and take time to have a conversation with them.

When it is not advisable to go out, we can do fun exercises at home. We can listen to music and dance. So what if we are the only one there with a client? Dancing is great exercise, and listening to music and reminiscing can be fun as well. This type of exercise is one way to keep our joints limber and our mind working. As a caregiver, we can dance with the vacuum. You will be surprised at how much conversation this will elicit. Again, we are loosening our joints and working our mind. Lots of people do crosswords together or play cards to keep their mind functioning. Although we can no longer get on the ground, and then get back up, how about a game of jacks or marbles on a game table or dining room table?

This is a great time to work on a new look for a part of the house. Maybe we want to have a corner of the living room dedicated to a hobby or grandchildren. Spending some time planning how and what we want to do is great thought-provoking fun. We move things into the area, look at them, and remembering when and how they became a part of us. This is also a wonderful time to put together some thoughts for our family to know more about us.

This is also a great time to start planning a garden. This is a good time to nurture our herbs and set up our hothouses. Setting up a map of our garden is good planning whether it is a vegetable garden or a rose garden. We can use this time to purchase seeds, bulbs, soil, and so forth at reduced rates. Also, it is a good time to plan and build raised flowerbeds or garden beds. This is a wonderful way to enjoy a hobby without stressing the legs or back.

Spring

Warm weather means several things; all of which will be fun and offer new sights and smells to our lives. We need to look at outside activities in two ways: what does this activity offer our daily wellbeing and is there a downside? Luckily, we will find more pluses than minuses to this time of year.

It is great for us to have a lunch and go out for a walk. Our food is used by our bodies far more efficiently, which will go far toward meeting our metabolic needs. It will also provide for muscle-building energy that will go far in the common battle with weight loss. These walks also provide stimulating conversation about plants and past adventures.

Our friend may be able to help outside and will

probably enjoy this activity. However, we must remember that our friend is still suffering from a debilitating disease and may need help with judgment and selection of the activities. Our friend should not be using the power mower or running a rototiller. Power tools are not part of the work anymore. Our friend may help in a supervisory capacity for activities that require these tools.

Planting in raised flowerbeds is a wonderful activity; however, you will want to watch out for any fertilizers or pesticides. Using a raised flowerbed for vegetables or fruit is a great idea and will allow for many hours of quality time spent together. Please be sure that you don't tire our friend out or over-stimulate them. These types of activities can be difficult for a tired caregiver to manage effectively.

Being outside—and with the weather getting warmer—it is time to once again look at the consumption of water. It is easy for our friend to become dehydrated in a very short amount of time. This is a problem that can be fixed easily and in a pleasant way. Of course, drinking water is the first and provides easy access. However, there are times when our friend will not want to drink water. We can add a small amount of lemon to the water to make lemonade; popsicles are another quick fix. We can get sugar-free popsicles so there will be no need to worry about any diabetic issues. We can add extra fruit to meet this need, specifically watermelon, grapes, and oranges.

If we are really eager to get into the nice weather

and enjoy spring, how about a picnic? This is easy to put together, and we will be able to enjoy the outside. We can stay at home, go out on the patio or yard, use own lawn furniture, or bring a household chair with arms for each of us with a small table. This will be great fun and allow for some different stimulating conversation. This can reduce stress for both of you.

Summer

Summer is a great time for enjoying early morning walks and harvesting some of the bounty from our garden. Fresh flowers are always nice to look at and smell. A secret to having flowers in a certain spot in our home is it challenges two senses and one memory process. The sense of smell is one of the first we lose as we age. In many cases, having cut flowers will help determine just how much loss we have in this department. The sense of touch is also challenged by how gently we can handle something. It is often difficult to feel the flower petals, and they get ruined. However, while this process is taking place, caregivers are able to get a clear picture of eye-hand coordination. And memory can be challenged by using timing stimulus with the flowers; what season are we in and what day did these flowers arrive in our home?

Although summer is a wonderful time to enjoy the outdoors, caregivers must keep in mind our friend's body will not adjust to changing temperatures as well as a younger person would. This makes our friend more inclined to get dehydrated in the hot part of the day and then not adjust well to the evening cool. Chilling can be a problem. When trying to keep our friend hydrated, water is the best tool. However, many people just don't drink an adequate amount of water.

Supplement with fruits containing large amounts of water; water-based drinks can leave a taste. Encourage drinking more lemonade or cranberry juice. Make popsicles and frozen fruit pops. Always keep in mind that with some medications, there are natural fruits and spices which are contraindicated. You can call your pharmacist and ask. Keep in mind that it takes a team to support our friend. We need to be careful that our friend does not have too much coffee or tea as these are dehydrating beverages. Alcoholic drinks are very questionable; they are dehydrating and can affect balance. We do not want any broken bones.

In summertime, more than any other time of the year, dressing in layers is beneficial. In the summer, it is cool in the morning and again in the evening. In between, the temperature can be toasty. Also, plan activities around this transition during the day. For instance, do not take our friend to the store in the middle of the day and leave them in the car while we run in for "just a moment." Invariably, we will run into someone who wants to know how our friend is doing. We could be away substantially longer than we thought we would be. Taking our friend to the marina or to a beach to enjoy the sights is a good outing for early evening or mid-morning, but we must be sure to take a light wrap. Watch body language for signs that our friend is getting cold.

The middle part of the day is perfect for staying out of the sun and being engrossed in a stationary activity, reading, looking at pictures, or listening to an audiobook together. Keep meals during the summer light and at room temperature. Hot, hardy soups or heavy meats and potatoes are more labor intensive than our bodies want to have for the most part. Having a half of sandwich with fruit or yogurt is a good meal; be sure that our friend gets the necessary calories during this time. You can always fill in with Ensure, Resource, or breakfast drinks made with milk.

This is a great time for lawn bowling or croquet if the yard is flat. Shuffleboard is another good outdoor activity to be played in the yard. The evenings are excellent times to wind down. Watching a moving or Super 8 home movies can be an excellent.

Fall

Fall is a challenge unto itself. If our friend has any dementia or difficulty sorting out what is real, caregivers are glad when this season is over. Not only are we trying to get outside activities put away and making sure that the house is ready for winter, but the stress of moving furniture and putting away planters and so forth is very hard for our friend to understand. Of course, they want to help us; give them some chores will boost self-esteem.

As Halloween items are put out in the store, if our friend can no longer distinguish reality from fiction, plan trips when we can take them—just not around displays. Distortion mirrors, displays that laugh as we walk by, or bursts of air or smoke can be frightening to some. Keep the candy away; these are empty calories and are not the weight we want. Just put one or two on the table and don't replenish that day. If our friend is having difficulty with this time of year, turn off your lights and don't answer the door. If truly frightened, we could be up all night, locking doors and pacing. This is just not the road we want to go down.

Past Halloween, we are going to start getting ready for Thanksgiving. If family members live close and are willing, the best bet is to ask what we can bring and then go to their house. And keep in mind our friend may decide at the last minute they want to go home. Should our friend decide to go home, discretion is best—just go home and visit another day. Our friend will not be ready for too much company and activity.

If we have elected to serve the meal, this will be an exercise in how well we can keep our friend occupied until a friend or family member arrives to entertain our friend. Do not feel badly that you are asking a visitor to help with our friend. Remember it takes a team to support our friend. If family is coming from out of town, try to keep the activity around our friend to a minimum. At the same time, allow the visitors to visit and see our friend on our friend's ground. One thing that never ceases to amaze me is how long our friend can hold all action and reaction together when company visits. Don't be surprised—just work with it and say, "This is a good day."

This is a good time to have the help we might need preparing for the upcoming winter. Casually ask a visitor to get the de-icer out of the garage up to the small storage on the porch. Or put the two twenty-pound bags of cat litter in the truck of the car for snowy weather. This is an excellent time to discuss the holidays that are just around the corner. Perhaps we have always had one of the days at our daughter's house and another at our son's; this may be a long, difficult drive. Try to establish a new routine; perhaps meet at mid-day and go out to dinner or have the family bring dinner in. Ask that all the gifts besides the exchange with our friend are done in advance to lessen the activity.

We can survive this time of year with a little forethought and cooperative friends and relatives.

Notes

Chapter 3:

Tagalongs

Please take the time to read these topics and try to prepare yourself in advance of the need. Each of these topics will impact your skills and your caregiving life.

What Shapes Us

Life experiences can become embroiled in caregiving. This is a coin with two sides. Our friend will bring to the table lifelong experiences that we may or may not know about. This can become especially difficult when there is more than one family history to sort through. If our friend has been married more than once, there may be different sets of children from each union. We will look at this scenario in one minute. Right now, let's look at the other side of the coin for life experiences of the caregiver. This is not easy for either side because each person's view of the situation is arrived at through this one person's remembrances, sights and sounds.

When we have multiple families, for the sake of our friend, communication is extremely important. If this is not the case, we need to look at the references we have. Have you played the game where everyone sits in a circle and an intentional play act occurs just outside the circle? Then we would start around the circle to see what happened only to find out that of the fourteen people sitting there, we have fourteen different events. Some differences may be more at odds than others, and some may seem quite similar.

Our friend may be suspicious of others telling or giving them things; their view has to be right. Unfortunately, this happens far more often than we want to believe. How we approach our friend is going to help us make the very best of this situation. As a caregiver, we must look at the situation as our friend does and see it through their eyes. Now we can explain it to them.

A good example is a sweet lady in her eighties who is living in an assisted living setting. A new caregiver is hired and begins work. Our friend asks the new caregiver to help her find her husband. The caregiver does not know the lady and cannot answer the need appropriately. The caregiver can say, "When I see you husband, I will tell him you are looking. While I do that, how about if you have a cup of tea at this table?"

The caregiver can go find someone to help out with the answers. Realistic answers will probably be that our friend's husband is deceased. Rather than telling her this, and having her relive all the heartache and pain, if she approaches us again, we say, "I haven't seen your husband today. If I do, I will make sure that he sees you right away."

She will probably keep looking; however, she is not as emotionally upset as she would be if we say he is deceased.

There are frequently times that we are unsure of the answer; when this occurs, do not lie. Always answer in generalities. If we are unable to find the answer, we should look for another avenue to try to find the answer, which may or may not be available to us. When we are working with a friend who has been married two or three times, the member of one family may or may not know the answer to questions that were taken care of in another family.

It is also important to know that it is okay not to have the answers. This is not a textbook situation, and the answers applicable in one situation will not be in another. The rule we must use is to do no harm.

Mirror, Mirror on the Wall

A phenomenon that happens frequently is our friend not recognizing the image in a mirror. Do not be alarmed if this happens, but be aware. Just as our friend is having trouble remembering people they have stored in their short-term memory, they do not remember that they are as old as they are. This happens frequently with progressive dementia. There are some things you can do to help afford our friend some peace within their own home:

- Cover up mirrors with towels or pillowcases.
- Take down mirrors when necessary.
- Keep shiny surfaces as dull as possible.
- Never leave our friend alone with a mirror in proximity.
- Do not try to tell our friend who is in the mirror; they will not understand.
- If necessary, invite the mirror person to join us at the table. Once we are all seated, our friend will probably move on to another exercise.

At this time, our friend will begin to confuse family members and friends. For example, a daughter may be mistaken for a wife or a son for a father. Our friend cannot distinguish the passage of time. This can be confusing when an old friend comes by with a son or daughter.

This is when inhibitions or social graces are no longer being followed. This will require our caregiver to be vigilant around other people. It is extremely important that we remember the actions and statements are being made by an individual who is ill. This behavior is not what we would expect of our friend when they were well.

Notes

Chapter 4:

Emotional Loss

Another loss that is particularly difficult affects everyone in the multiple roles surrounding the person with Alzheimer's. The only good thing you may say about this loss is that it does not significantly affect people suffering other dementia.

This loss is the one of self. Our friend may lose the knowledge of self, not recognizing themselves or others who have played significant roles in their lives. This loss is especially hard for spouses and children of the affected person. Imagine a spouse who has been married to our friend for more than half a lifetime. They have shared births and deaths of immediate family, as well as dreams, wants, and desires. Imagine an adult child living in close proximately for a lifetime. Perhaps they carried on the family business. They also shared dreams and learned to navigate the world from this person.

Imagine our friend not recognizing the spouse

or child. Or they believe the daughter is our friend's wife or the son is the husband. This seems so foreign, but it happens daily in dementia care centers for Alzheimer's patients and other dementias. Imagine how hard this would be to live through each day as a home caregiver.

Our friends are doing the best they can in the world they have been given to live in. Each family member and caregiver is also doing the best they can. There are very few things that can be done to make this situation any better; it is what it is. What we can do to help our friends and the caregivers is to listen as they express the pain they are going through (don't try to take it away; listen and empathize). Be available to give these caregivers a break (for them, it can be overwhelming). Be compassionate to our friend. There is so little that friends and family can do—and that is a loss for all concerned.

Caregivers should rely on a network of help. Don't forget there is respite care in most communities. Know where respite care is and how to access it quickly. As a caregiver, you must take care of yourself. Otherwise, your ability to help and be available is decreased dramatically.

Caregivers should seek help for every question or turn in the road. Don't try to manage all by yourself. This is a long road that will require work, caring, advocacy, and tears.

Communication

How many times have we seen a couple or been part of a couple when words were not necessary? We know the emotion behind the smile or eyes. How many times have we eaten a meal or seen a picture and known what our partner was thinking without either one saying anything.

Doctors, nurses, counselors, mothers, and fathers have always said, "Use your Words." Perhaps it is not the best way to help someone if you must try to communicate without words, but it happens every day—thousands of times. The key is to do accomplish this delicate dance without agitating or frustrating the person who is unable to speak.

Speech therapy helps the communication happen. However, we don't seem to use these tools as much with the elderly. Perhaps there is good reason for this lack of education. If a person has a medical problem, it will not allow them to retain the knowledge. Why can't someone help those of us who care for the person affected by the problem? If our person is not able to use a picture board to show they want food, why can't we be taught to help them with other tools?

We return to the concept of knowing your friend. If the life pattern has been for this person to stay up at night and watch late shows, then sleep in until 9:00, why would we expect this person to get up at 6:30 and eat breakfast in the dining room? If the life pattern for a person is to have coffee and read the paper after dinner, why would we put the person in front of the TV and leave them there for two hours? This scenario happens every day in structured living arrangements. If this were us, wouldn't we want the courtesy of being a part of our lives?

Communication is not nearly as difficult if we stick to the known life patterns of our friend. Of course we are not going to know the answer every time. When a person is generally a sweet, gentle soul with few demands and no outbursts, what do we do when the opposite becomes true? The first thing is to make sure they are not being hurt. Hurt can be pain or fright. If these do not appear to be the problem, try to establish when the initial demonstration was.

If the initial demonstration was at the dining table, check the dentures. Could something be wrong with them? Is a piece of food under them? Are they someone else's dentures (it happens in facilities more than you want to know)?

Was the initial demonstration at the bathroom? Does this person have a history of bladder infections? When you have gone through everything you can think of and anything anyone else in the caring group can think of and you are sure the person is not frightened or hurt, try playing soft classical music, lowering the lighting, and keeping the area quiet. You will be surprised by how well this will work.

After all else has failed, we add prescription drugs to the mix. Our elderly friends with dementia do not metabolize medications well. Many do not drink enough water, and their bodies are in constant flux or adjustment.

Physical Touch

We go through our daily lives and don't give thought to how many people we physically touch each day. However, for the elderly and disabled, there is very little access to people outside their small world. And if that world is made up of professional staff and one or two friends, they either don't receive any physical touch or very little. We are physical in all we do during our life, and there is an emotional deficit when that is taken away.

We must have physical touch in our lives. The lack of this touch is devastating to our physical and emotion wellbeing. The emotional lack of stimulation will lead to a physical cascade of health-related issues.

If there is no family present—or they do not want to accept this responsibility—this need falls to caregivers. Many of us do not have a clue how to proceed without leaving ourselves open to legal problems. However, we can accomplish this in a professional way without creating a problem. Always ask for permission prior to touching our friend. Until you know this person well, respect their private space (imagine a two-foot circle around them). Always get an invitation prior to reaching inside this space. Getting an invitation or permission will keep out any miscommunication between us and our friend. Even when shaking hands, we extend our hand, leaving it out far enough that the other person has to extend their hand to shake hands.

A therapeutic hug is one where only the shoulders touch; it lasts only a couple of seconds. Full-body hugs or leaning over our friend to hug them are too intimate and can cause confusion. When leaning over another person, we are the dominant person, which is setting up disaster in a caregiving relationship. Giving a full-body hug may lead to unwanted or unwarranted advances and emotions.

Touching the top of a hand as we are leaving is a great way to say I will return. Say good-bye and pat the top of the hand a couple of times. This will ensure that our friend has had some human contact and provides knowledge that we care and respect our friend.

One way to ensure human contact is to give a hand massage. This is a great way to build lines of communication with our friends and affords necessary human contact. If our friend is in a coma or unaware of the minute-to-minute activities around them, touch or rub around the temples, speak softly, or play a CD of nature sounds.

The most important thing to remember is that we are here to provide professional comfort—not unnecessary stress. If we are professional and remember good manners, there should not be any misunderstanding.

Pain

We touched on how to know if a person that cannot communicate in words has pain. Let's go a step further with what caregivers can do. Pain is a very elusive medical diagnosis.

Since it is so difficult to determine pain as causation for actions, caregivers can use a small amount of time to eliminate other causes. Has your friend always had a level of pain? Many people in our culture live with pain on a daily basis. It may be from a physical diagnosis related to employment or genetics.

Our friends do not stop having pain as they age. Having knowledge of how our friend lived is a great barometer of pain, whether treated now or in the past. Many of our friends may live with pain and choose not to go into detail with us regarding this topic. An excellent example is a military veteran who served the required time and then was discharged. During the active duty time, our friend was in an automobile accident and hurt his back, causing lifelong pain. Although, we may never have discussed this with our friend, military information may be available to help us—or specifically our friend's physician.

If we knew our friend prior to them being unable to communicate, it is prudent to sit down and talk. Learn what you can for a medical and social history while you can. This will provide us with many aspects to help our friend. Many memory care centers will have a staff member sit down with family, friends, and the new patient to gather this information. This history will be invaluable when trying to determine medical matters and help our friend feel more comfortable in day-to-day living.

Should we come into the situation without considerable knowledge of our friend's history, we must begin to put the puzzle together. Although this may seem futile, keep in mind our friend deserves all the compassion and caring we can bring to the table.

Some of the best ways to help our friend, in the absence of prescriptions, is to meet the emotional need. This can be as simple or as intricate as you want to make it. Begin with soft lighting—still vision-supportive, just not glaring light. Use no sound, soft music, or nature sounds. Keep the sound level soft, almost as if you were walking in the forest and there was no traffic. If our friend accepts touch, gently rub circles at the shoulders and base of the neck (always with clothes on). Always ask permission before touching a friend. If no sounds are being used and we feel comfortable doing so, we can hum. This can be especially relaxing, and our friend may fall asleep. Remember to only rub the soft tissue of the shoulders and neck. Sometimes, a better way of reaching that emotional peace is with damp, warm washcloth or warm rice pillows. If utilizing this comfort mode, be sure that the water or rice is only slightly warm to the touch. As people age, the skin becomes sensitive. If we are not careful, the skin can burn. We should treat the skin of an elderly person as we would treat that of a newborn.

While pain is difficult to diagnose for a person suffering from dementia, so are other emotions in life. Frequently, emotions are out of context and cannot be explained. Our friend may cry while watching an old comedy. We simply need to acknowledge the emotion they are experiencing.

Do not make a great deal—or ignore—this emotion. Just treat our friend as you would any friend who suddenly experienced a raw emotion.

Exercise

Caregivers don't have much time for taking care of their own needs. Many don't even consider trying to get to the gym. There seems to be little we can do to accomplish this—and we are tired and just want to sit down. However, we have had little glimmers of light when there has been a chance to exercise. What can we do?

One great way to add exercise to our day is to take long walks. When we go to the grocery store, park at least ten cars deep in the parking lot (this is, of course, without our friend). Take our friend to a hardware store or fabric store to walk; this is good for both for us. Join the mall walkers in the mornings when our friend is up for it.

When time allows, take a fifteen-minute walk, journal, and read. We will get the benefit of walking and relaxing. When we walk like this, we should put all of our emotion into it. Step hard on this walk—as if we are using this time to get rid of the frustration of this curve life has thrown at you. This is excellent self-care.

Dancing is great exercise, and dancing with our friend is a good exercise and activity. Dancing can be done while we are doing housework; a vacuum will work just as well doing the salsa as the routine back-and-forth motion. The music is a good way to rejuvenate our bodies and relax us. The music will help our friend with balance and strengthening back and leg muscles. We can have fun—who can be unhappy when dancing?

If that inner baker is trying to get out; why not bake bread? Don't use a bread machine; get into that flour up to our wrists, knead the dough, and work it every hour. This is excellent exercise for our arms and upper body, but there is nothing better than the smell of fresh baking bread to motivate our friend to eat.

Recently the YMCA has added a "River Walk" which is great exercise for both of us. This is a graduated slope in an S-shaped portion of the exercise pool. The water goes to four feet deep; a gentle current pushes against us and provides some resistance. This is great exercise and will provide stimulation for our friend (www.ymca.net/find-your-y).

We can always have a specific day and time for going to the gym. Coordination of caregiving responsibilities is the key. Most trainers recommend a set routine so that the visit will not be put off. This can be our personal time. Providing excellent self-care and stimulation with other people is so important. If we find the time and want to check out a local gym at little or no cost, there are plenty. Research local health clubs or check this site: www.aarp.org/member-benefits. It is essential to check with our doctor prior to beginning any exercise program.

A Sense of Self-Worth

We all want to be productive members of our own household. Most people have worked and provided for others in one way or another. Many people have spent much of their lives volunteering to help others. Now they must let someone else do things for them—from a small amount of help to meeting their most basic needs. This lack of involvement can cause depression and a lack of value. This is especially true of older adults who have retired and then spent several years volunteering.

We can meet this need with some out-of-the-box thinking. If you have known our friend for a great amount of time, you will probably know what gave our friend the most self-esteem in their lifetime. If we are just meeting our friend, we will have to look for this catalyst and put together some home projects to help our friend feel of value again. This may sound easy, but you are going to work hard at this task. However, it is going to be one of your greatest moments in caregiving.

First, look for work or activities that have filled

our friend's life with self-esteem. Do their pictures show some cherished moments in life or do plaques commemorate their milestones? Take the ideas and visualize providing this idea within the caregiving environment. While doing so, you will create two important ideas for our friend.

- Our friend still is a contributing member of society and has value and worth to themselves and our community.
- You will provide a reason, a feeling, and an idea that leaving this place will not be as good. This action will decrease wandering outside the home. We have just provided what they are looking for.

There is a way to accomplish this task and get a few minutes to rejuvenate our batteries. If our friend volunteered at a food bank, ask the management of the food bank what our friend can do to help them out for an hour a few times a week. There is always something: opening bags for the clerk to put groceries in, entertaining children while their parents pick up and load groceries, or restocking cans.

If our friend used to write manuals for pipefitting, find an old typewriter and desk. Stock the desk with paper (typing, lined, and graph), pens, and pencils. Take our friend to the local hardware store for supplies and ask the clerk if they have some broken or unusable pipe. (You have just accomplished two tasks:

the beginning of a self-esteem project and helping our friend get exercise.) Pull out tools and other items for our friend to use while writing the manual and let them go to it.

I know you will find more ways to help our friend, but remember we want to boost their self-esteem. You will have to adjust this from time to time and find new roles for our friend, but you are on your way.

How to Encourage Our Friend to Take Pills When Necessary

This can be the most daunting task when there is little or no cooperation. Before long, we are frustrated and bordering on angry. There are several ways of handling this situation; however, do not keep trying until everyone is in a bad mood or angry. We are here to help our friend—not to do everything for them. Tell them in a mellow but firm tone to take the medicine. If it doesn't work, ask them to take the medicine while your body language and tone indicate you are asking for their help.

Do not stand over our friend; sit beside or in front of them. Don't push the medicine; this will only cause you more problems in the future. You can check the mechanics of eating and drinking for our friend; has there been a change or a grimace while eating or drinking? If so, our friend could have a sore throat or another medical problem. Check for fever. If they have dentures, check them. If this is not the issue, our friend just does not want their medicine; leave the issue and come back to it in fifteen or twenty minutes. Continue to try through lunch. If you are making no progress and they really need to take their pills, try putting them in a small amount of ice cream or applesauce. If this problem continues, our friend should go to the doctor.

Did you know they make almost every medicine in liquid form? Most of the time, the pharmacist can give you some ideas for how our friend should be taking the medicine. There are medicines that should not be given with some foods; be sure to ask the pharmacist about this issue.

Notes

Chapter 5:

Medical Needs

Advocacy needs are in this world as important as having a physician who knows your medical history. If you go to the hospital or doctor's office, you will be asked if you have a Medical Durable Power of Attorney (DPOA).

The physician or multiple physicians will want and use this document if we cannot answer for ourselves. There are multiple reasons why we may not be able to answer for ourselves (surgery, medications, or an accident).

Our lifestyle will determine who we want for a medical advocate. It is wise to have an alternate should the first advocate not be willing or able to answer for us. We, of course, will talk with our advocate at great length about our desires and wishes in different medical situations, but who's to say we won't both be in the ER at the same time due to accident or illness. The person we pick should most certainly be someone we are sure will be willing to assert our wishes—even if these wishes are not what our advocate would choose for themselves.

This is a difficult and stressful position to be in. It is also one of great honor and an unsurpassed expression of faith in our advocate's character. When we choose a family member, friend, legal advisor, or a paid case manager, we will need to meet several times to be sure that we have expressed our values in life and expressed wishes should there be a need to decide about quality versus quantity. We should be sure that our advocate will be able to meet the direst of situations with a clear mind and strong heart.

There are pros and cons to whether you select a relative or not, but it is important that the individual will be able to express our wishes. (I know lawyers whose wives will not give them DPOA because of such a strong division of beliefs.) Bringing in a friend or sibling is a matter of choice; it is always a good idea to give careful consideration to any disagreements we have had in the past. A paid case manager is one way around family issues, but how well do you know the ethical and professional background of this person. Just because it is something we are paying for does not mean our wishes will be met. Check carefully on backgrounds and ethical issues in their professional lives.

Another important part of our planning is to make sure that all persons know who the advocate is. Make sure we provide the physician, lawyer, and next of kin with the appropriate paperwork to clarify our wishes. All our hard work is for naught if the people who need to know are not in the loop.

Use this table to track behaviors and the unusual situations. You may find it of great help as you look at the Global Deterioration Scale on the next couple of pages

Behavior	Connection	How Often	Safety Risk	Frequency

Global Deterioration Scale

GLOBAL DETERIORATION SCALE (GDS)		SCORE
Level	Clinical Characteristics	
1 No cognitive decline	No subjective complaints of memory deficit. No memory deficit evident on clinical interview.	☐
2 Subjective cognitive impairment	Subjective complaints of memory deficit, most frequently in following areas: (a) forgetting where one has placed familiar objects; (b) forgetting names one formerly knew well. No objective evidence of memory deficit on clinical interview. No objective deficits in employment or social situations. Appropriate concern with respect to symptomatology.	☐
3 Mild cognitive decline **(Mild Cognitive Impairment)**	Earliest clear-cut deficits. Manifestations in more than one of the following areas: (a) patient may have gotten lost when traveling to an unfamiliar location; (b) coworkers become aware of patient's relatively poor performance; (c) word and name finding deficit becomes evident to intimates; (d) patient may read a passage or a book and retain relatively little material; (e) patient may demonstrate decreased facility in remembering names upon introduction to new people; (f) patient may have lost or misplaced an object of value; (g) concentration deficit may be evident on clinical testing. Objective evidence of memory deficit obtained only with an intensive interview. Decreased performance in demanding employment and social settings. Denial begins to become manifest in patient. Mild to moderate anxiety accompanies symptoms.	☐
4 Moderate cognitive decline **(Mild Dementia)**	Clear-cut deficit on careful clinical interview. Deficit manifest in following areas: (a) decreased knowledge of current and recent events; (b) may exhibit some deficit in memory of ones personal history; (c) concentration deficit elicited on serial subtractions; (d) decreased ability to travel, handle finances, etc. Frequently no deficit in following areas: (a) orientation to time and place; (b) recognition of familiar persons and faces; (c) ability to travel to familiar locations. Inability to perform complex tasks. Denial is dominant defense mechanism. Flattening of affect and withdrawal from challenging situations frequently occur.	☐

Stage	Description	
5 Moderately severe cognitive decline **(Moderate Dementia)**	Patient can no longer survive without some assistance. Patient is unable during interview to recall a major relevant aspect of their current lives, e.g., an address or telephone number of many years, the names of close family members (such as grandchildren), the name of the high school or college from which they graduated. Frequently some disorientation to time (date, day of week, season etc.) or to place. An educated person may have difficulty counting back from 40 by 4s or from 20 by 2s. Persons at this stage retain knowledge of many major facts regarding themselves and others. They invariably know their own names and generally know their spouses' and children's names. They require no assistance with toileting and eating, but may have some difficulty choosing the proper clothing to wear.	☐
6 Severe cognitive decline **(Moderately Severe Dementia)**	May occasionally forget the name of the spouse upon whom they are entirely dependent for survival. Will be largely unaware of all recent events and experiences in their lives. Retain some knowledge of their past lives but this is very sketchy. Generally unaware of their surroundings, the year, the season, etc. May have difficulty counting from 10, both backward and, sometimes, forward. Will require some assistance with activities of daily living, e.g., may become incontinent, will require travel assistance but occasionally will be able to travel to familiar locations. Diurnal rhythm frequently disturbed. Almost always recall their own name. Frequently continue to be able to distinguish familiar from unfamiliar persons in their environment. Personality and emotional changes occur. These are quite variable and include: (a) delusional behavior, e.g., patients may accuse their spouse of being an impostor, may talk to imaginary figures in the environment, or to their own reflection in the mirror; (b) obsessive symptoms, e.g., person may continually repeat simple cleaning activities; (c) anxiety symptoms, agitation, and even previously nonexistent violent behavior may occur; (d) cognitive abulia, i.e., loss of willpower because an individual cannot carry a thought long enough to determine a purposeful course of action.	☐
7 Very severe cognitive decline **(Severe Dementia)**	All verbal abilities are lost over the course of this stage. Frequently there is no speech at all - only unintelligible utterances and rare emergence of seemingly forgotten words and phrases. Incontinent of urine, requires assistance toileting and feeding. Basic psychomotor skills, e.g., ability to walk, are lost with the progression of this stage. The brain appears to no longer be able to tell the body what to do. Generalized rigidity and developmental neurologic reflexes are frequently present	☐

The Global Deterioration Scale for assessment of primary degenerative dementia. Reisberg, B.; Ferris, S H.; de Leon, M.J.; Crook, T. The American Journal of Psychiatry, Vol 139(9), Sep 1982, 1136-1139. Copyright © 1982 Barry Reisberg, M.D.. Used with Permission

Global Deterioration Scale
Draft version one

Reisberg, B., Ferris, S.H., de Leon, M.J., Crook., T. The global deterioration scale for assessment of primary degenerative dementia. American Journal of Psychiatry, 1982, 139: 1136–1139. Copyright © 1983 by Barry Reisberg, MD

Smooth and Seamless Medical Appointments

It's one thing to have the time and thought preparation for a scheduled appointment. It's entirely another to have a quick trip to the urgent care or emergency room. We can help make this go more smoothly than thought possible.

First, we need a copy of all pertinent information upon arrival at this type of appointment. The most important information is covered by medical information: Medical Durable Power of Attorney, current medication list, a current list of all allergies, contact information for the medical provider, a brief medical, and reason for the appointment. Truly, this is not as overwhelming as it may seem.

We must remember only to provide current copies. Sometimes copies of information get lost, so we will keep the originals. In a folder, place a copy of the Medical Durable Power of Attorney on the right flap and contact information for the immediate medical provider (also on the right). On the left side (in this order from back to front), include medical history, current medications, and allergies. The reason for specific information on the right or the left of the folder is if we walk in on a situation that requires immediate de-escalation from us or in a life-threatening situation, you will only need to hand the file to the physician or RN in charge. They will immediately recognize the importance.

Make a second folder with the same information.

Place both folders in your automobile in a safe place with easy access for you to grab them automatically as you go into the emergency room or urgent care.

Having this information on hand will help us concentrate exclusively on the immediate needs of the person we are caring for. It will give the medical professionals addressing the care a glimpse into the medical life of our friend. They will see us as the knowledgeable, caring person we are.

These folders will require little management. The only page needing to be changed regularly is the medication list. At different times, we may need to change out the Medical Power of Attorney, but everything else will only need minimal adjustments. This can be kept up without intruding into our everyday life.

There are several reasons for having two folders, but the biggest reason is if you need to change between urgent care and the emergency room or between hospitals, you will have a backup available.

Sundowning

Sundowning is a term given to the unique behaviors that seem to become more prevalent in the late afternoon or early evening and will sometimes last well into the night. The behaviors, as you can well imagine, are not calming or providing a feeling of safety. Actually, they can be unsafe and dangerous.

Sundowning usually includes paranoia and

frequently will create a fight-or-flight situation within the person's environment. This frequently is the case when the person has lived in the same dwelling with the same person or people for many years.

There are many thoughts of how to best undertake providing for the person's safety. The most common and immediate is medication. While we are looking at the issue of safety for our friend, family and/or caregivers, medication is foremost in everyone's best interest. Once the situation is under control, it is an immediate concern to look at the overall effects of the medication and the environment.

There are several ways we can provide for our friend in a safer and calmer situation. This may be the time when caregivers and family want to decide on a more structured living situation. Professionals find that, at this time, the spouse or caregiver is living in more of an unsafe situation than our friend. They may get little or no sleep out of concern that our friend might leave the home or become abusive of the caregiver. Every possible safety mechanism has been put in place to protect our friend. However, when all medications were put away and out of reach, the caregiver's medications were too. The caregiver is now working on little sleep and making sure that our friends has taken their medication. But did the caregiver take their medication? Maybe they should take it now?

Keeping our friend inside at night can mean installing locks that we would never think of using otherwise. When someone needs to get in the house, our friend inside can't provide a much needed service. It can be difficult without professional help. Although I would hope this has been done prior, please get all weapons out of the sight and reach of our friend. This includes all firearms, knives, machetes, solvents, lighters, matches, and so forth.

This is a difficult subject and should not be taken lightly. You are not alone or in a quagmire of lost hope; there are answers. You are just stuck in the mud right now.

Supplying medical information can be frustrating and embarrassing. Our friend is continuing to lose independence in large pieces. Perhaps one of the most stressful losses for our friend is not having doctor-patient confidentiality. We each have the privacy that is shared only with our clergy or medical provider.

Our job as the caregiver is to facilitate this independence for our friend without jeopardizing their welfare. A variety of tools can provide this communication with confidentiality. Your first step is to bring the medical provider into your confidence. Most times, the provider will thank you and help you find ways to get the necessary information to them. This transfer of information may be by telephone, e-mail, or notes given to the receptionist or nurse when checking in for an appointment. Once the information is in the provider's hands, we can rest assured that you have provided the best available appointment. It is important to remember that more and more medical professionals do not use English as their first language.

Things we will want to pass on to the medical provider are changes in our friend's ability to take care of themselves, issues with incontinence, seeing or believing in people that are not there, an increase or decrease in appetite, a change in sleep patterns, or new actions or beliefs that concern us. Something as simple as dehydration can dramatically change behavior.

Some of us are caregiving for friends living in a nursing home or residential care outside of our dwelling. Please still be involved and attend those medical provider appointments as much as possible. We are still the best resource your friend has.

The way to have seamless, best outcome with a medical provider is to have an open line of communication. This is especially important if you live in an area that adheres to the hospitalist (medical provider in hospital only) model. Be sure to know what medication our friend is taking, what they are eating, and how they are acting. The hospitalist, in all likelihood, has never seen our friend before and will only be involved for a short amount of time.

Frequently in this model, the medical provider will receive calls to gain some insight into the friend, but as more and more medical institutions are connected by electronic records, much of the information is readily available.

Notes

Chapter 6:

Legal

Caregivers, by nature, focus all attention on the friend they are working with. After all, isn't that why we call them caregivers? Sometimes, caregivers need to look at a much bigger picture.

Particularly for family caregivers, there is a real need to look at legal documents early in the picture. This can also be true for paid caregivers since they sometimes look at a much larger arena of events. When our friend or patient is ill—and this is going to be the case for some time—there are many decisions to be made. This is a particularly stressful time, and it seems the cup is running over with decisions to be made. This is especially true with respect to legal decisions.

You are already familiar with the decision regarding the wellbeing of your friend or patient. And should you not be in the know as to what documents you need, soon you will be overwhelmed with requests for them. The most important are the Medical Durable

Power of Attorney, the Financial Power of Attorney, and joint rights to bank accounts and finances to defray cost of this illness and later on to the executor of the estate and so forth.

What is generally not discussed at this point is if there are any legal documents that our friend or patient is the holder of power on. To be specific, is our friend the Durable Medical Power of Attorney for a spouse or disabled adult? This legal state needs to be passed on to another person as an instrument of their power and responsibility. If possible, the decision maker in this situation should not be the same as the person making decisions for our friend or client. The emotional weight is overwhelming for one person, especially if the person is a parent.

Our friend or patient is unable to legally act for another individual because they are just getting by themselves. The most common case is a husband and wife who determined the need for these documents long before either was ill, and the one with the disease is the custodian of legal permission to act for the well-being of the other well one. There is also, more frequently, the case of an ill friend or client having legal custodianship of an adult with a significant mental impairment.

When asked if our friend or client has a Medical Durable Power of Attorney covering anyone else, a relative will say, "Yes. I hadn't thought of that." Some attorneys do not think to ask the question. The thought process is so narrow, encompassing only the individual with the illness, that the other persons are lost in the work being done to safeguard the ill person.

It may seem foreign or outside the question, but the senior population is growing exponentially. Due to advances in medicine, many children born to the aging population were not given a long life expectancy. Many were given up immediately—or almost immediately—and later returned to the parents or family (brothers, sisters, aunts, or uncles) due to the cost of providing care for them. And now our friend or client who has held the legal documentation for all these years is ill and incapable of making decisions. The first cases to come to mind are a parent of an adult with Down's syndrome and a parent with an adult relative who has sustained a brain injury. As we look at the family dynamics, we can see other situations needing the same relief. There is even the case of our friend or client having the legal instruments for a father or mother and our friend or client being diagnosed with a terminal illness.

This heart-wrenching situation has slipped by, and we are in a situation where the decision maker is incapable of making the necessary decision. There are two possible outcomes: our friend or patient is led by family or medical personnel into a decision the well person believes to be in the best interest of the emergent patient's case or the patient is placed on life-sustaining protocol and a medical ethics team or a court must make the decision.

Neither of these situations is acceptable from an

ethical or familial point of view. However, they are cases in our current medical community.

Caregiving is a difficult job for a paid caregiver, family member, or friend. If we can get some help, it is a good thing and a wise choice. Talking about end-of-life decisions and concerns is difficult for everyone; however, it is an important topic to be familiar with. As we go about our business of caring for our friend in medical, financial, or dual roles, it is important to keep the end-of-life issue within our sights.

Do we know what our friend wants concerning their end-of-life care? What does our friend's family want? What is our doctor looking at for end-of-life care? If our friend is in a facility, what is their role in the situation? Every one of these entities is just as important as the other. If we are unsure how to approach this topic with our friend's family, there is a great little tool called "Five Wishes," which we can use to get the conversation going.

If we are the spouse and caregiver, it is even more important to check with immediate family members and make sure that everyone are on the same page. We frequently find this is not the case, and our friend becomes the object of a family struggle. Most of the time, this is because of the finality of the situation for no reason besides the contemplation is so distressing to our being. And as we have more and more blended families making up our communities, there will be more room for opposing views. This goes to the reasoning that family should have many communications during life as to what each wants in a given circumstance for medical care and final wishes.

Please consider this even if you are a young adult with the best health and do not foresee any reason for this conversation. That sentence is probably the best reason for having the discussion. Who is to say you will not have an automobile accident or be shot on a street coming out of a cinema. It is important for adults who would be making decisions for you at that time to know exactly what you want. Gone are the do-you-want-to-donate-your-organs days (we as a nation have done a superb job of getting that topic out there). These are the days of life support and sustaining life at all cost regardless of the quality of life after. And if this life is saved and this person is in need of exponentially invasive care for the rest of their life, who will be there as the person's advocate, financial advocate, and Durable Power of Attorney for medical needs?

There is no right or wrong answer, but it is the time to have conversation and know that if called upon to make any decisions we will make the decision our friend wanted in this set of circumstances.

It is important to know your state's laws and regulations surrounding the decisions you are making. Twenty-nine states accept Five Wishes as legal documentation if signed by our physician, including California, Washington, Idaho, and Alaska. There are differing views regarding this issue; don't get caught up in this part of caregiving. www.agingwithdignity.com

Notes

Chapter 7:

Living Where — Our Choices

Do we really have choices as we age? We have choices in almost all decisions and aspects of our lives and how we live. The dilemma is how and who will look or research the choices for us. We have never had as many choices as we do now. We have never had to look for answers as we do now. We have always had our choices provided by medical providers, clergy, and family. In many cases, family lives hundreds of miles away. Medical providers have passed the baton for living choices to social workers and case managers. Clergy members are focused on a smaller population than in the past.

To understand what has happened to our ability to see our choices, we need to understand where our choice helpers have gone. Clergy members are not as close to families as they have been in past generations. Before, clergy members would know family members by name and would have a cursory knowledge of what our choices might be in a life-altering condition. At the very least, they knew where family members could be located. Due to a generation of moving away from organized religion and for many other reasons not communicating with local clergy, we are adrift in a sea with many other people. Although, it does appear that the current generation is moving back in the direction of seeking advice of clergy.

Medical providers have moved in their relationship to patients from being adviser to providing medical treatment of a cutting-edge quality. We are probably expecting too much of these human beings. Medical providers are rarely general practitioners today; will send us back to whichever provider gave us the consultation with the specialist. This is like roulette wheels that we pop out receive treatment for one symptom and then get back in the game. However, there is no home place where all the autonomy and values are held to guide our medical practitioners. Family is in the four winds due to lifestyle and economic reasons. Certainly, there may be some family issues at root, but even when none are there, it is crossing a bridge for family to get together and help one another.

We must find our own advocate to help circumvent the social, medical, and financial needs we may face. Clergy is probably the easiest of the three fixes for us to accomplish. We will need to reconnect with this part of our advocacy. This may not be as easy mentally for us, but it will be easier than connecting with our medical provider. If we have a medical provider who is acting as a general practice physician for us and is not going to retire before we need these services for aging, keep them close. This is a rarity in today's physician/patient relationships.

For the first time in history, we are outliving our medical provider's practice. Doctors retire, become ill, or look at all the chaos in the medical field and chose to leave—prior to our aging bodies needing their services. Our choices are relatively slim: get a new, younger doctor, look at other physicians within our physician's medical office and determine if they will be there at the time we need, or continue with the knowledge that many hospitals have hospitalists now. Most Skilled Nursing Facilities have their own medical officer.

Family is an area that would be better left to each person. If we believe our family will be there for us at that moment of need, keep them apprised of your medical decisions and concerns. Make sure they know of our health care desires. For the first time in history, our decisions will be brought up and questioned and advice sought aside from whether you want CPR.

Medical technology is so far advanced past the CPR question that we now find our medical personnel asking for medical directives. We definitely want our medical decision maker to know our wishes and have our best wishes at heart.

Structured Living

Sundowning and dementia care specifically require some thought about what is needed in a place for our friend to live. Many Americans in need of help, but who are still able to walk and feed themselves, do not need go to a Skilled Nursing Facility (SNF) or nursing home. There are other choices, but the choices are not equal. To begin our search, we need to determine what care and support our friend needs—and what kind of support we need.

Does our friend wander? Does our friend want to leave on their own? Does our friend require a special diet? Are we concerned with diabetes, low sodium, or allergies? How many medicines does our friend have? How many times a day? Can our friend dress themselves?

These are and most important. When we look at resources in our community, it is important to take a tour of the facilities (assisted living or adult homes) without our friend. Everyone has different tastes and concerns. That being said, if there is a strong dislike on our part, there probably will be our friend's part too. The move to a facility will not work if we are distrustful or do not like it. The benefit of touring can be undone if we take our friend. Our friend may become suspicious or paranoid.

Once we have found the facility we like best, we need to speak with the person whose job it is to intake new residents. Begin with your most pressing concerns.

They might be money (the cost of services), wandering, leaving our friend, or stepping out the door.

One cautionary tale regarding cost is that there will be a base rate—and then there will be points for care or ancillary services or added services. That is where the monthly bill will grow unexpectedly. Just be aware and ask questions; you will find layers of services and amenities. There are also places to save money. We might want to continue doing our friend's laundry or using the same pharmacy to pick up and deliver own medications to the facility.

Other questions or concerns may come up as you go on this journey. However, they will provide a good start. With them in mind, you have an opportunity to begin this process without the situation driving the train; you will be in control of the train.

Moving into a facility providing care can be very difficult. There are many ups and downs associated with moving for the elderly or disabled. First and foremost is the loss of independence—whether real or perceived. For many, this is the first step into a nursing home. It would seem—to younger, more able-bodied folks—to be a misjudgment. However, for our friend, it is just one more loss at a time when they are losing significant parts of themselves. Now they are, in their own minds, losing a home and a car at the same time. They will not have the choice about what they eat, when they eat, when they bathe, or when they go shopping. Some of this is true, of course; much is an expected backlash from the move.

How can family, caregivers, and friends make this easier? First and foremost, allow as many decisions as possible to be made by our friend. This may add time to the moving process, but it is better spent now than in the weeks and months ahead. Try to put plans in place to allow some independence. When you are to visit, call and ask if it is convenient. You would do this when our friend lived in their home and drove themselves—stick by that courtesy. It will not fail you.

If you help with shopping, let our friend pick the brand and or type of purchase. Let our friend invite you over—even when it may be inconvenient for you. This is a way of taking ownership of their residence.

Most of the time, it is not appropriate to take our friend to live in a residence where they have not had a choice and we have already set-up for them. Even when our friend is at the hospital and will need to leave the hospital to live in a care facility, we need to provide for their ownership of this new home—temporary or not. When dementia is involved, we can help setting up a room for our friend, driving them, or meeting them as they are brought from the hospital.

This is exactly what some structured living facilities ask. This is, they say, to create less stressful moving situations. Please evaluate this for our friend and make an informed decision regarding your situation. Helping with the physical move is appropriate, even necessary, but helping with the selection of what to take or how to decorate the room is usually something that we can do together. If our friend is moving due to a recent fall or illness and is weak, begin the planning while they are in the hospital. Allow everyone to take part in helping our friend, but be sure that permission was asked and thank you was said. If time permits, use a diagram to make decisions about where to place larger items in the room.

Even when suffering from a disease or mending from surgery or a fall, our friend is still the person we have known and loved. When dementia is involved, you will have to be a little more creative in helping our friend making decisions. Allow some help making the decision to move, begin the conversation with a question regarding an earlier time in our friend's life. Move slowly and deliberately through the discussion you have planned out prior to the meeting. Always allow the decision to be our friend's while using their input.

With short-term memory loss, our friend will forget the decision was made. However, if approached right at the time and then going back using positive, loving conversation, our friend will be able to own the decision again.

Adult Family Homes

Adult Family Homes (AFH) are just as the name suggests. Houses within the community are licensed by DSHS to provide caregiving support to persons unable to meet all their physical and mental needs in their own home. These needs can be anywhere from not remembering to call 911 in an emergency to being unable to prepare food or not meeting any of their ADLs. There are state laws that cap the kind of care provided; however, if the home is licensed as having an RN on premises and is acting in the proper manner, they can provide care for most anyone not needing the most invasive medical care.

Many AFHs are as specialized as Assisted Living Facilities. Some will provide only the minimal care necessary for helping our friend through their day. Some will be open to having hospice provide end-of-life care within their walls.

The important thing to determine is whether this home can provide care for our friend—and for how long. While most AFHs are licensed to take only a set number of residents (four to six), the staff is usually educated only to a certain limited level. There is a loving and honoring care provided in AFHs. However, if we are looking for an AFH for our friend because we can no longer care for our friend due to dementia and paranoia, we should give this a great deal of thought and look strongly at assisted living. Should there be six residents with two caregivers and one of the caregivers does not show up, one caregiver who is taking care of our friend and five others.

AFHs can be the best placement in the world for a person who is aging gracefully in their own setting but is starting to fail due to small, mounting issues.

They will always provide a more stimulating environment and be able to meet individual needs (special menu items, laundry, entertainment, and so forth) far beyond other facility care. Illness and medical needs seem to be caught quicker in this setting than in most others. AFHs are respectful, caring places for a population not requiring day-to-day nursing care. Many older Down's syndrome folks live this lifestyle with the absolute best results, unencumbered by rules and larger populations of Assisted Living or Skilled Nursing Facilities.

Although families are in the driver's seat for this part of the care, paid caregivers should be looking at this situation as well—partly due to the stress this will bring to the patient and partly because a paid caregiver is there for the patient and the patient's family is also part of this case.

Skilled Nursing Facilities

Skilled Nursing Homes are the last of the structured living settings we will look at. SNFs are not the stark, sterile ones from the fifties and sixties. Today many hire interior decorators and enhance atmospheres with a variety of home-style solutions. There are many that appear as a three- or four-star hotel as you enter. Other SNFs add to the homey feel with pets and plants.

The other idea you will need to embrace when searching for placement is that 95 percent have a specific focus for the placement of patients. Some

SNFs have a specific focus on physical therapy, surgical rehabilitation, invasive medical treatment, or dementia.

If our friend has fallen and broken a bone, the physician will want physical therapy after surgical intervention. It may be recommended that you seek a SNF that focuses on physical therapy. A patient suffering from a strong dementia possibly will not do well in this setting. Too much stimulus and paced therapy are overwhelming. The second piece of this placement is that a staff that has been specifically trained to work with physical therapy is not necessarily able to include dementia care. Also, many people with dementia do not learn new techniques well.

You will find the same problem in a SNF trained in dementia care. This is when you will need to guide the placement very carefully and with thoughts clear of what is best for our friend. There are many physicians who work from the medical model and have difficult thought processes surrounding placement of an individual with dementia.

Our friend should be given every opportunity to recover; however, this may not be with physical therapy. We are the holder of the knowledge in the case of our friend. We must look at the setting and decide if it would be better to have them reside in a dementia-care SNF with in-house physical therapist coming to see them regularly. A person will make a better recovery if they are less stressed about daily life.

The next part of the task is far more difficult. When do we acknowledge that our friend is not going to be able to continue with any certainty of improvement? This is usually decided by the physical therapy team; once our friend goes to a SNF for this reason, a timeline is put in place. Medicare will only pay for one hundred days of therapy if the individual is making progress. There must be charted progress for our friend to continue to receive physical therapy being paid by Medicare.

Notes

Chapter 8:

Finances

Finances play a role in every type of medical issue. It is important to know that a physician will as if a specific treatment is *really* what our friend would want if treatment is available, but will not have life-enhancing effects. We need to be prepared for difficult questions a physician, nurse, or friend may ask.

At this point, it is important to take financial account of where we are and where we are going. This is a difficult topic to discuss, but it is important to approach it. If you know the finances and the direction this illness is taking, you can budget for the most appropriate outcome. Unfortunately, this is an inevitable part of the care to be provided. When we look at the cost of medical care and the benefits available, our job switches to being the person with the purse strings safeguarding our friend.

This is the why many lawyers and courts like to

see one person in charge of the finances and one person in charge of the medical matters. As we look at all the concerns, we may want to split the duties.

Financial Information

Let's talk about the economics of lengthy illnesses. Many who carefully planned and saved for retirement are in financial straits. This is the most expensive part life for an aging population, and it happens to be the largest population in terms of retirement and the financial future of our nation. A point of interest is that the graying parts of our society have more difficulty getting jobs than any other group in the nation. However, this group needs medical care and resources that they thought they were paying for as they worked and contributed throughout their adult lives. This is not a political statement—just a fact.

You may not be aware of certain monetary lifelines. The population we are talking about was the generation which objected to our military involvement in Viet Nam. However, if you were in the military at any time of war (even if only for one day and you were in the US at the time), you are eligible for some benefits. Please do not assume that just because you chose an alternative to carrying a gun, you are automatically not eligible. Also, there are certain forms of employment that have benefits you may be unaware of.

The railroad, mining, shipping, and marine services all provide benefits we have yet to apply for. Of course, federal employment provides some benefits. There is a very clear pattern of benefits that is paid out at the state and federal level.

An overwhelming amount of information is coming at us from the medical, financial, and family arenas. If we can sit down for one visit with a person who knows these benefits, it will be an enormous amount of help. The quickest way to find this person is to look in your telephone book for federal, state or county agencies that focus on the elderly and disabled. It is unfortunate that, with all our resources in this country, we do not have a clearinghouse with all the information available to us.

The Area Agency on Aging and Long-Term Care will be able to help us find many of the answers; however, they may forget to remind us that our property taxes can be discounted substantially by contacting the tax assessor's office and filing some papers (remembering that our property was our fall back if all monies ran out). If you live in an area with a large federal employment base, contact the local employee benefits advisor.

Washington has a group called Columbia Legal Services, a wonderful resource for financial eligibility for programs at the state and federal levels. There is even more information available at http://apps.leg. wa.gov/wac. There are places for the safeguarding of funds for the surviving spouse, and there are ways the well spouse can keep the house for the length of time they remain living there. There are local service agencies that can help with utility bills and in some cases with cash. There are Meals on Wheels to help with food at little or no cost.

We have just scratched the surface of the help that is out there. It seems a shame that we don't have a better way to get the information out to those in need. Many areas have begun the use of a telephone triage or clearinghouses for some of these services. Begin with your local services and then move on to federal services; there is some help—we just have to be willing and able to look for it.

Notes

Chapter 9:

Other Important Issues

There are some very important topics that have a force and definition of their own. I have included them in this section to allow you to have some forethought should you want to—or have to—consider them. Some topics will make your heart skip a beat and then race forward; others will make your heart smile.

Driving

Americans associate their ability to drive and ownership an automobile as something akin to a coming-of-age right. We drive everywhere. For the most part, we look at any mass transit as something the other person does or if the car is absent for a few hours or days. Most of the industrialized world views driving as a luxury. When a person has dementia, driving becomes a weapon. It can do as much harm to the driver without hurting another person as any other weapon.

A car is a challenging piece of equipment that

can be used to take us to the store or get us so lost in the maze of vehicles and buildings that we are frozen in fear. We do not do our friend a favor by allowing the driving to continue when the reflexes are no longer adequate. Would we allow our friend to use a chainsaw when they are too frail to hold it up and too confused by all the buttons to let go of the trigger? Our friend has trusted us to help them through this part of their life because they believed that we would know when to say enough is enough.

Taking the keys is probably one of the hardest things we will have to do. Our friend very possibly will be angry and hurt initially. We can help our friend and remain a friend by talking to the doctor or e-mailing the doctor ahead of an appointment. Many doctors will take on this task when they realize the enormity of the situation. If not, the highway patrol or state patrol will be able to help by inviting our friend down for relicensing. Some of our friends are really in the know and are willing to give up driving. This is a good reason to disable the car or have the driver's license put away. Many people will not drive without their license or insurance.

You are doing this for them—and not *to* them. Our friend would not want to be driving if they were able to view the whole picture. Please do not think they can drive to the store if you send the phone with them. Once our friend is lost, panic exacerbates the confusion. Our friend would not want to be a statistic—that is why they have asked us for help.

Caregiver Stress

Caregivers frequently have significant health issues, especially when the caregiver is providing care for a family member. Since women have held the caregiving roles within families in larger numbers than men have, we see more women with significant health issues—even death.

Caregiver stress frequently leads to depression; it is prevalent in times of health care issues, financial upheaval, and family discourse. Depression does not seem to affect more women than men when the ratio is caregiver to non-caregiving roles. It is obvious that stress and depression rely on each other. Part of this comes from family make-up and part comes from education, rather than gender.

It appears that the best way to combat depression in this scenario is compassion and support. We are a nation of individuals looking for the easy fix to a very complex problem. Popping a pill is not a long-term answer. If appropriate information and education are given to this issue, the prescription will be more compassion and support—not a chemical change within the body.

This is not a simple solution, and it is not one to take lightly. Our friend's needs are overwhelming and the person, more often than not, already has health issues that were only mildly under control prior to the onset of this caregiving situation. In many cases, women are looking at lifelong caregiving, which is a 24/7 role, or they have been focused into a career that is leaning on the guilt of not being present at the onset of the illness. Men have corresponding roles, frequently being away from home and focusing long hours in a job they may not have had a passion for or wanting to be physically involved in the caregiving process. However, their only role can be working to provide health insurance.

Many physicians and human resources representatives have not educated our caregivers about the Family Leave Act of 1993, and then taken up by the Department of Labor for enforcement in 2006. The resounding theme was guilt. Interestingly, guilt is one of the stages of grieving. We have layered grieving for self to grieving for a close family member.

As we see, there is no easy answer, but we need to begin taking care of ourselves at the very beginning of caregiving. Set up some rules and build in some personal time on a daily basis. It can be a ten-minute meditation, having a chart so we drink eight glasses of water each day, or exercising while we do our other work. We just need to build these things into our days. Later, build a half or whole day into our week; this will allow us to really recharge our batteries. Attending a support group may sound like a bad use of time, but consider it one of your most valuable tools. You will have the opportunity to hear from others who are in same place as you. They may offer you a tip you had not expected.

This is the very tip of what is going on with

our caregivers; however, we can help them make a tremendous financial dent in elder care. Support of the caregiver needs to be right at the beginning of the illness and medical care for the affected person. We need to recognize and provide support for our caregivers through access to social service programs, education of how to take care of themselves as well as the person affected by illness, and ongoing supervision and escalation of support needs for the caregiver. This program of support and compassion needs to be ongoing and increase as needs evolve during the length of the illness.

The American Institute of Stress has some revealing facts that correspond with information from the Mayo Clinic. Not all stress is bad, but we have to manage our stress when it comes to caregiving. Although many kinds of stress require medical intervention, caregiver stress needs far more advocates and social service networks to help with stress relief and taking care of self.

Pets: Where Do They Fall In All This

Seniors with pets are the exception to the rule; when people age in place, a shrinking of the safety net is inevitable. With our new research and education about how we age, having pets is important. There has been an ebb and flow with respect to who is there for the elderly when help is needed. However, the pet is devoted to the person through thick and thin.

The aging community depends on pets more than children in many cases.

The young elderly (30 to 50 years of age, keeping in mind that early onset Alzheimer's Disease can start as young as 30) seem to know how to best provide for themselves without the intervening of family. However, as we continue to age, we have not yet summoned the expertise necessary to help us continue this evolution. This is another reason why we see pets becoming more and more of a lifestyle for us. Looking at where we choose to reside, it is immediately known that if people can choose, they will choose places where they can take their pets. The bond between people and pets comes close to the companionship of family. We want our pets to be with us; they have served as confidants, friends, providers, and family. Many people live great distances from family; this is an opportunity to not feel so alone.

As we age, there is a continual passage of losses. It starts with the loss of friends and acquaintances. This gives rise to the daily loss of hearing, sight, and independence. Losing a driver's license is one of the most difficult losses for the elderly. While their parents may not have even had the opportunity to drive or own a car, we have become prisoners of the industrial age. The loss of the ability to drive is surpassed only by the loss of a child or spouse.

Armed with this knowledge, senior living solutions have policies in place to allow our seniors bring their pets with them. This is just one more sign that pets can be a vital piece of the aging process. Seniors who have and care for their own pets live longer and happier lives. Pets help us to continue living productive, useful lives. Having a pet and keeping it can be the difference in thriving and existing. We need to foster this kind of cohabitation since it provides less expensive and less overall health care.

Activities

Many activities will help you enjoy your time together in a constructive way while allowing you to become closer to our friend. One activity is to massage hands or feet. It is simple and pleasant for both parties. Let's say we are going to massage the hands. Get a dish of warm soap and water (use a small dish with warm water and dish soap). Place the hands in the warm water and allow them to get warm (be sure you have brought a dish of plain water to rinse the hands and a towel to dry them). After the massage, it is refreshing to use a light lotion with no fragrance to rub gently on the hands and wrists.

Once the hands have begun to warm up, take one hand at a time. Gently hold the hand and rub it with your thumbs. Gently rub in circles to feel the skin but not to move it. As this is taking place, talk with our friend about past travels or other pleasant experiences. You might want to discuss a shopping trip where our friend purchased a specific piece of jewelry or clothing that meant a lot to them. You might want to discuss a picnic where the weather was warm and the scenery was especially beautiful. If you are the spouse, you might want to reminisce about the marriage proposal. A child might want to ask if our friend remembers a specific school play, Halloween costume, or wedding dress. Any of these would be very respectful topics, which would make it a meaningful, pleasant experience.

Another nice relaxing experience is to create an inside picnic. This is easily done with the use of a table and chairs (no getting on the floor or trying to get up is more like it). Light finger food and soft nature sounds from a CD allows an experience without concern for falling, bad weather, and so on. This is especially nice if the outdoors have played a significant role in our friend's past.

None of this should be romantic; they should be reminiscent of past experiences. This will allow our friend to have a quiet, peaceful time without the worry of why things are not quite the way they should be. If you are a paid caregiver and are wondering how to approach this, try inviting some of our friend's family over to help with the event and station them between you and our friend.

Mirror, Mirror on the Wall

Our friends with dementia might finish this line with mirror, mirror on the wall, who is that anyhow? It is hard to imagine but in a progressive dementia—Alzheimer's, Parkinson's, Huntington's, or Lewy Body Disease (www.mayoclinic.com/health/lewy-body-dementia)—patients do not recognize themselves. As hard as it is for us to imagine, consider what it must be like for our friend. What can we do as caregivers when faced with this reality?

The first thing we must realize is that mirrors are not all equal. The mirrors you know are mirrors can be taken down or covered up. However, there are times during the day when shadows and lighting can turn a glass cover on a picture mounted on a wall into a mirror or a TV screen. When you walk into a room with a half-glass entryway, we understand. The windows on our homes can become a wall of mirrors. How do we compensate for these mirrors that are out of our control?

One of the best solutions is to have a plan in place prior to the need. In many cases, we can know about this problem in advance. Watch for the behaviors at home and begin the planning at that time. Walk between our friend and a mirror to break up the reflection. Make sure that our friend is not facing a mirror. Make sure that helpers are aware and know the triggers and solutions. And never argue with our friend about the image they believe is before them. Talk about the situation or the emotion they are experiencing. Remember our friend is having an experience that is their reality. Afford our friend the same grace and humility that we would afford any other person.

The ramifications of such phenomena can be disastrous. Our friend may choose not to use the facilities in the restroom if there is a stranger in there. Our friend may not disrobe for a bath or shower for the same reason. One of the worse cases, for me, was a man who refused to eat because his friend (in the mirror) was not being fed. This is not an easy thing to fix once it becomes a habit. It is not funny and should never be treated as such. Our friend truly believes that there is another person in the room.

The thing that makes this easier to work with is our ability to change pathways at home or in public. It is important to keep in mind that these episodes are called hallucinatory events. People in other walks of life with no prior medical history of dementia may also suffer from this, but the treatment will be entirely different. Our friend is at a point in life when medications seem to muddy the waters of illness and may actually be worse than the disability. At this point, compassion is the better part of valor. After all, this is our friend's reality.

Holiday Celebrations

Our friend enjoys eating, visiting old friends, smelling holiday smells, and other nuances of the holiday season. This is a time of over-stimulation for individuals with dementia or other chronic illnesses. Rather than being a time of joy and happy memories, it is very stressful.

Many times, the caregiver will notice that there is less food being consumed. Our friend seems all right; it is not another illness, just a lack of appetite. Any time of year can add stress to our friend's life and daily rituals. However, this time of year seems especially difficult for our friend. First of all, there are so many more things going on. Everyone says, "Happy Holidays." Baked goods are coming through the door, and there are many new smells. Christmas trees may be trimmed, family is coming in from out of town, and maybe some are staying at our friend's house. This is a lot for someone who is not ill to handle, but this is like putting the last drops in the rain barrel for our friend.

The key to helping our friend is to simplify everything we can. Maybe the company could come by to visit for a shorter amount of time with different folks coming at different times, allowing two or three hours to rest in between. Perhaps those folks intending to stay with our friend can stay with someone else or keep their activity to a minimum around our friend except when it is their turn to visit. If it has been a family tradition for the family to gather in one place, suggest that, rather than multiple conversations around the room, singing Christmas carols would be less frustrating for our friend.

Try hard to maintain the usual routine. When eating, especially in a group setting, limit the choices on our friend's plate. Depending on how confused or stressed they are, limit the food choices to one or two.

Do not limit the amount of food—just the choices. If they really like potatoes and gravy, serve a small portion. Keep an eye on the food; if the potatoes and gravy are gone, ask if they would like some fruit salad. Always be sure that they have enough food to eat, but keep the choices down.

The same can be true with visitors. Try to keep the numbers down. Explain the need to keep the commotion down in a jovial manner. The giving of gifts can be an exciting event, but it can be stressful for our friend. Suggest the adults go out to a fun meal to catch up. Have one family at a time come in to exchange gifts.

Gifts for a person who is ill can be an interesting experience. The idea of giving a picture of the family when they were younger or an album or scrapbook is wonderful because it allows for interaction with our friend. This type of gift can be very meaningful for everybody. If the caregiver comes into the family after the time of making a gift of pictures or scrapbook, what insight the caregiver will get.

We must realize our facilitation is much more than housework, bathing, eating, and going to medical appointments. We are the helpful bridge between what has been and what is. We need to help our friend enjoy the season without the strain of the season. We only to be caregiver, social director, custodian of medical information, purchaser of gifts for our friend to give, traffic controller, and chef, to name a few.

Simplifying the eating process will become more

important as time goes on. If you need a break, let a trusted family member or friend put on your hats for a couple of hours. Do something for yourself—you deserve it.

When the holidays are over, we are exhausted and so are the people we care for. This would be a good time to reflect on what has been. For our friends suffering from Alzheimer's, we could reflect on holidays, childhood memories, and times of joy. For our friends who do not have short-term memory loss, focus on well-remembered times. Dementia is only one reason we are here to provide care. Reflecting on what has been for anyone ailing from an injury or disease provides a way to re-establish his or her self-esteem.

Self-esteem is a significant factor to help people move forward with their lives. Being productive and useful is better than being sick and uncomfortable. Quality is what most of us want as we move forward.

This is a great time to have someone help clean the house and take down the holiday decorations. If money is tight and hiring someone is out of the question, contact your local Scout organization or high school. These students have a set amount of volunteer work they must do, and many see the writing on the wall. As students will tell you, adults looking for employment are holding many volunteer jobs, but this is a foot in the door. These groups are generally well supervised and instructed on proper work manners.

Perhaps we want to know these people better.

Start our education now for spring yard work that will be difficult to tackle. Having a project like this is a win-win for both parties. If you are a member of a local church, let them know. This is another way to get help after the holidays.

Volunteers bring new conversation, ideas, and different faces to boost the self-esteem of our friends. Volunteers—no matter the age—provide a new picture for our friend. One of the volunteers might visit with our friend while we explain what we need done and where. What a blessing that would be for all. Self-esteem and quality of life comes in many different packages.

Notes

Chapter 10:

First Aid for Caregivers

Be prepared to take charge of life's little obstacles when you are a caregiver. When there is no one to call, we need to take the bull by the horns and move on. One of these times is when we get up in the morning for a full day, find out it has snowed four inches during the night, and learn the extra help we were counting on will not be there. These sorts of things happen to all of us; however, if caregiving is our primary role, they are especially intrusive.

You are not alone. Although it sometimes seems like too much is happening, you will rise up and meet this head on. I know this because I have been where you are right now and have barged through it. I hope I can bring some grace to how you will approach and handle these challenges.

Caregivers need summer time for themselves, but there isn't a lot of time for caregivers to take a few days off. If these are paid caregivers, they have vacation time from their employment agency—and a substitute is sent to help out while they are on a vacation. What happens when the caregiver is a family member?

Family and friends frequently do not get time off while they are in the thick of things. Unless the caregiver mentions it, others simply do not think of it. Most do not see this as a need for caregivers or realize how hard it is for them to get away. Frequently, adult children offer a vacation getaway for Mom and Dad, feeling that they have done something thoughtful and nice. The trouble is no matter which one is the caregiver, the caregiver is going to be carrying a lot more weight. We all know the extra things we have to do to go on vacation; it seems like a lot of work, but we have others helping and happily sharing the work. Our caregiver does not have that; they have a friend who is worrying about why new, misunderstood things are happening.

When our friend has dementia, one component is paranoia. This can create a circle of fears and behaviors. Caregivers are trying to get mail stopped or picked up by someone, making sure there is enough medication for the days they will be gone, making sure all necessary food items are taken care of, and packing and loading luggage in the car. Once they have reached the destination, the work must be repeated as they prepare to return home. Frequently, during this time, our friend is confused and feels unsettled, causing more work for the caregiver.

Is it any wonder caregivers in the front lines do not wish to take vacation? If you are a family member of a caregiver, this is one birthday or early Christmas present you can give that will be much appreciated. Maybe there is a family reunion coming up; this is your time to really be of help. Help the caregiver by helping out.

The caregiver might say, "I just don't know where to start?"

Make some suggestions that you can accomplish to help. Then help get the work started; be there every step of the way for the caregiver and friend. Once there, start giving the caregiver quality time to do things themselves. When it is time to leave, provide all the same help you did when getting ready for this trip. Stay and help get everything settled, making sure there is food in the house for three days, the mail has been picked up, and there is plenty of medication for our friend. If you have time, help get the laundry done and the first meal on the table.

You may think this is not really a present or a place for you to be involved, but you will see and hear tenfold how much help you are. For some, this comes naturally, but for many this is a new side of life. Meet this new frontier head on and you will be rewarded.

Extreme Weather, Extreme Stress

After periods of extreme weather, take a day to go out and take care of yourself. We are thinking about all the things we should have, could have, would have—but the truth is we did the very best we could at that time. We were the one there, and we did the best we could. So let's de-stress and rejuvenate. Take a long walk or go to a quiet place to let everything go. Get back to being healthy and feeling good. Caregiving is hard work. If a weekend is necessary to help put everything right in our body, soul, and heart, then that is what needs to be done. Respite is your safety net.

When all this is behind us, we have relaxed and are moving on. Let's sit down and journal what we can about the experience. Our journal is not for others to read; keep it safe and handy. After a month, analyze what we did, what we could have done, and how we will handle this next time. Let's make all this stress work for others and us. It may seem as though we have enough to do without providing guidance for others. However, nothing will help us stay healed on this rocky path we walk better than bringing our knowledge and experience to others.

You are aware of the selfless giving and caring necessary to help our friends who are struggling. I take off my hat to you for a job well done. More than anything, I know this is not a job to you—it is a calling. Congratulations for the selection of a calling that will serve you well as you help your friends

Getting prepared for a disaster or local emergency may sound foreign and overwhelming; however this is the time. We are preparing for at least two people—and one is going to have a significant hurdle to get over. Each county has a disaster preparedness official who meets the needs of residents—young, old, disabled, living alone, or in a community residence. The focus is on the disabled and elderly, which is a very large population—and it is growing every day.

We hear frequently about being ready for the Big One, but where do we start. The Department of Emergency Management will have guidelines for you. If they do not, this is the time to remind them. They should have lists of provisions and shelters set aside for this population. There are some intrinsic needs developed for this population. They will have to address medication management, special dietary needs, level of cot to floor, personal hygiene for incontinence, and how to get information to families quickly.

Our job will be to set up a disaster kit for three days and medication for two weeks. Our disaster kit for three days should be set up as though we are the only help for our friend during these three days. Purchase a kit from the American Red Cross www.redcross.org or make a kit from lists on the website. Look up emergency preparedness kits on the Internet. Not all emergency preparedness kits are equal, and caregivers have enough to do. The Red Cross has been doing this job for many years; they are experts.

Another important task to remember is keeping the medication in prescription bottles with the correct prescription from the pharmacist. We have to visit this part of the kit every time there is a change in medications. This may seem cumbersome, but it is necessary. Once our friend is in the shelter, a designated nurse or EMT will take over the medications. They need this information and will not deviate from the prescription. There should be a letter in the kit explaining the general health problems of our friend and who the doctor is.

If we are relying on paid caregivers, they may not be able to get to our friend. Tell neighbors or someone living close by about the location of the emergency kit. This will afford time for someone who knows our friend to get to them.

Check where the closest shelter for the elderly and disabled is. Be sure that those needing to know that information do know. When we change our clocks and check our smoke alarms and batteries, call to find out if there has been a change in the location of the shelter.

Notes

Chapter 11:
End-of-Life Thoughts

I do not pretend to know your circumstances or how to handle them, but at some point, we will all have to face this prospect. And if this should happen without forethought, frequently there is regret.

There are no answers here, but I have stood where you are and have had to make difficult decisions. I came to the decision arena with some knowledge and preparation—thanks to medical professionals and clergy. I hope you will have the opportunity to fully consider all avenues and make decisions based on knowledge and expertise—not misunderstandings, fear, and lack of knowledge.

Caregiving is a difficult job—whether it is as a paid caregiver, a family member, or a friend. When we get some help, it is a good thing and a wise choice. Talking about end-of-life decisions and concerns is difficult for everyone; however, it is an important topic to be familiar with. As we go about our business of caring for our friend—in the medical, financial, or dual roles—it is going to be important to keep the end-of-life issue within our sights.

Do we know what our friend wants for end-of-life care? What does our friend's family want? What is our doctor looking at for end-of-life care? If our friend is in a facility, what is their role in this situation? Each of these entities is just as important and vital as the others. If we are unsure of how to approach this topic with our family or friend's family, Five Wishes can get the conversation going.

If we are the spouse and caregiver, it is even more important that we check with immediate family members and make sure that everyone is on the same page. We frequently find this is not the case, and our friend becomes the object of a family struggle. Most of the time, this is because of the finality of the situation and the contemplation is so distressing. As more blended families make up our communities, there will be more room for opposing views. Families should have many communications during life about what each wants in any given circumstance for medical care and final wishes.

Quality versus Quantity

The question of lifestyle and beliefs will very possibly come up at some time during your caregiving duties with other providers, medical professionals, and family. I am not here to give you the answers; the only one who can truly answer it is our friend. In absence of our friend's ability to vocalize personal wishes, this question will fall to whoever has the Durable Medical Power of Attorney.

If you are the person this power of medical decision has been bestowed on, I would suggest you begin putting together your knowledge of the wishes of our friend. This question historically has been made between the physician and the patient with family being advised. However, with the medical advances and family living at great distances, information gathering is difficult at best.

Although the question may never be utilized due to illness and living situations, you will be asked in many ways anytime our friend goes to the hospital or a new structured living setting. The question could come up again if our friend is returning to a structured living setting.

At the very least, it is a difficult question to answer. *If your heart stops, do you want CPR? If you should fall gravely ill, do you want all medical means available to be used to keep you alive?* These questions have been grounded in our health care system for many years, but never to the extent as they are today. Everyone is weighing in on this subject, and it can be difficult to determine the answers. The more information you have, the easier it is to understand the wishes of our friend.

Most people have outlived the practice of their primary care provider. Hopefully the new physician has all the medical information regarding end-of-life decisions, but do not count on it. Many specialized physicians only impact a small part of our friend's life—and no one is the keeper of the knowledge.

If our friend has dementia, can they understand the gravity of the situation? Can they explain the life-sustaining measures they want? Our litigious society has made this question even more difficult since many physicians do not want to take on this responsibility. If the planets align and our friend's best wishes as known to everybody, but our friend says the opposite of what was everyone's understanding, it sets the legal system in motion. "Do no harm" will be followed and, until a higher power can be consulted, this is the road we shall go down. This road will be driven without respect to cost, family wishes, or prior documentation.

Our knowledge is what will save the day. Our friend believes we will protect and serve his or her wishes—that is why we were chosen. This is a daunting responsibility, but we have been blessed with it by our friend. We can liken this responsibility to that of a godmother, godfather, and friend in the truest sense of the word.

Each of us has specific beliefs or customs that we expect to be present or addressed at the time of our passing. These are the core of who we are. Some will say they want to be left alone and not make any noise. Some will say they want family with them at the end. Some will want clergy or medical staff with them.

We are the keeper of the flame—unless otherwise specified.

We will have the information and must be willing to help facilitate last wishes. Maybe our friend wants to be outside in the sunshine with head tipped back and facing the sky. There are ways we can help this happen without flying to Arizona. This set of beliefs is more basic than food and water; it is as important as the breath they take.

Solve this problem prior to the need to activate. Make sure any family that may be present is aware and understands the last wishes of our friend. The facilitation we are about to do is at the request of our friend. Rarely is there any question by family; however, this is not the time to have it, if possible. There will be no do-over, it must be right to start with. If you feel that you cannot accommodate these actions or beliefs, please search for another who can.

Throughout this book, we have discussed parts of life that make up who we are. We have discussed the need to look to someone who is strong and will support the wishes of our friend when difficult decisions arise. This could not mean more than it does with end-of-life questions and concerns. Our nation is struggling with major financial issues; these issues will come to rest on the largest aging population in our nation's history: the baby-boomers. We have always lived in a comfortable state of knowledge that our medical needs will be met. This is simply not true anymore. We are in a downward spiral; the medical needs of our citizens are outweighed by the sheer numbers of the population. We must begin planning and preparing for the rainy day of limited care.

This is not a forecast of gloom, but it is a prediction of needs. We have fought hard and won the battle to have an end-of-life solution of hospice. This has been provided in Europe for many years, and we see the need for this care within our borders. With the financial decline of our social service programs, the medical field is looking to a new specialty of palliative care. The goal is the same; however, there is a world of difference financially.

Hospice is funded under a federally subsidized program that will not cost the recipient anything. This was the philosophy behind the need for this kind of care. A hallmark of this care is that the recipient has six months or less to live. And although they do not hold a a firm line, that is the expectation from the beginning. This funding has more to do with funding of the program, and the physician's assessment of the persons condition than anything else.

Palliative care is provided to the receipting that will allow for the person to move along in their disease process with the expectation of the most comforting of medications, therapies, and treatments. The financial side of this is that your health insurance will need to pay for this, and your payment for the care is not covered.

They share a common goal, but the means to the goal are extremely different. Looking at the financial and health insurance make-up of our population, it can be conceivably said that our next add on to Medicare will be "Part Z-End-of-Life Care." If we are the decision makers for our friends, it is falling on us to be sure that there will be paid end-of-life care.

What will our plan of action be?

Notes

I hope that this book has added some stability in the otherwise storm of caregiving. I wish you all the best as the road ahead of you is one filled with potholes and detours, yet beautiful sunrises and shocking clarity.